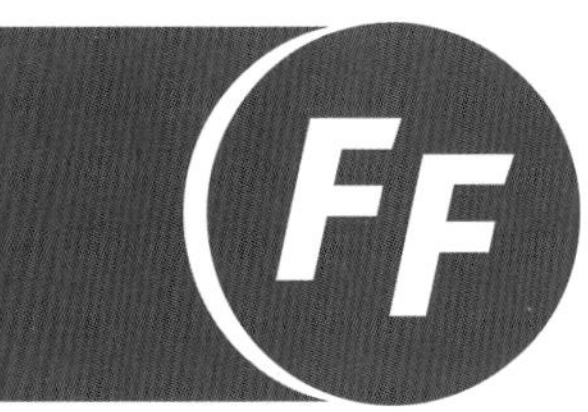

Indispensable Guides to Clinical Practice

Dyspe

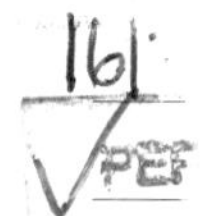

Second edition

Kenneth L Koch
Professor of Medicine and Chief,
Gastroenterology and Hepatology,
North Carolina Baptist Hospital,
Wake Forest University,
Winston-Salem, North Carolina, USA

Michael J Lancaster Smith
Consultant Gastroenterologist
and Director of Research and Development,
Queen Mary's Hospital,
Sidcup, Kent, UK

HEALTH PRESS
Oxford

Fast Facts – Dyspepsia
First published 2000
Second edition January 2003

Health Press Limited, Elizabeth House, Queen Street, Abingdon, Oxford OX14 3JR, UK
Tel: +44 (0)1235 523233
Fax: +44 (0)1235 523238

The authors acknowledge the excellent secretarial assistance of Pamela Petito and Kerry Sharpe in the preparation of the original manuscript.

A CIP catalogue record for this title is available from the British Library.

ISBN 1-903734-19-3

Koch, KL (Kenneth L)
Fast Facts – Dyspepsia/
Kenneth L Koch, Michael J Lancaster Smith

Illustrated by Dee McLean, London, UK.

Typeset by Zed, Oxford, UK.

Printed by Fine Print (Services) Ltd, Oxford, UK.

Glossary

Achalasia: a condition in which the normal muscular activity of the esophagus is disturbed, delaying the passage of swallowed material

Achlorhydria: absence of free hydrochloric acid in the stomach

Barrett's epithelium: columnar cell lining of the esophagus instead of normal squamous cells, induced by chronic acid reflux. It is associated with an increased incidence of cancer

CLO test: test for *Campylobacter*-like organism, the old description of *H. pylori* before it was reclassified

Cox-1 / -2: cyclooxygenase-1 / -2

Dysphagia: a condition in which the action of swallowing is difficult to perform or in which swallowed material seems to be held up in its passage to the stomach

EGG: electrogastrogram, a recording of the myoelectrical rhythm of the stomach

Eradication treatment: pharmacological therapy that aims to eradicate *H. pylori* from the stomach. Most commonly used regimens comprise a proton-pump inhibitor and two antibiotics, given over 7 days

Esophagitis: inflammation of the esophagus usually due to excessive exposure to refluxed gastric acid

Gastroparesis: paralysis of the stomach resulting in delayed gastric emptying

GERD (GORD in the UK**):** gastroesophageal reflux disease

LES (LOS in the UK**):** lower esophageal sphincter. Normal LES pressure is 12–40 mmHg

MALT: mucosa-associated lymphoid tissue

Meckel's diverticulum: a pouch in the wall of the distal ileum; it is a congenital abnormality

Nissen fundoplication: the most commonly performed surgical procedure for GERD; the gastric fundus is wrapped around itself and the distal esophagus and any hiatal hernia is reduced

Odynophagia: pain on swallowing, rather than a burning sensation rising into the retrosternal area

PPI: proton-pump inhibitor

Torsade de pointes: tachycardia in which the electrical stimulation of the heart undergoes a cyclical variation in strength; it gives a characteristic pattern of twisted spikes on the electrocardiogram

UBT: urea breath test, a non-invasive test for establishing current *H. pylori* infection

UGI: upper gastrointestinal

Zollinger–Ellison syndrome: condition characterized by excess production of gastrin usually due to a G-cell tumor of the pancreas; this leads to hypersecretion of gastric acid and ulceration of the esophagus, stomach, duodenum and jejunum

Introduction

The term 'dyspepsia' defies precise definition, but is generally understood to mean symptoms suggestive of upper gastrointestinal (UGI) disease (Table 1). Symptoms associated with changes in bowel habit or defecation are excluded from the definition of dyspepsia and are classified as components of irritable bowel syndrome. Dyspepsia may be caused by many conditions, including diseases of the pancreas and biliary system, but the majority of patients with dyspepsia have an organic or functional disorder of the upper alimentary tract (Table 2). Heartburn and regurgitation have such a strong association with gastroesophogeal reflux that they are now excluded from the classification of dyspepsia.

Dyspepsia is extremely common in Western society, with a prevalence of 25–40% over a 6–12-month period. Only 25% of sufferers consult a doctor; they do so not only as a result of symptom severity, but also because of concern about potentially sinister disease.

Although dyspepsia accounts for approximately 5% of family physician consultations in the USA and UK, only a fraction of patients are referred to specialists. In the UK, for example, only about 10% of patients with dyspepsia are referred for specialist investigation. Despite this, annually 2% of the UK population undergo UGI endoscopy or barium-meal examination.

Although in most cases dyspepsia is the consequence of benign disease, it is the cause of significant reduction in the quality of life.

The economic consequences of dyspepsia are impressive. In the UK, nearly 9 million prescriptions were written for H_2-receptor antagonists

TABLE 1

Symptoms of dyspepsia

- Upper abdominal pain/discomfort
- Anorexia
- Early satiety
- Bloating
- Nausea and/or vomiting

TABLE 2
Definitions of dyspepsia

Organic dyspepsia

Symptoms due to specific abnormalities that are confirmed by diagnostic tests, either:

- morphological (peptic ulcer, gastroesophageal carcinoma, esophagitis detected by endoscopy) or
- pathophysiological (esophageal reflux detected by pH monitoring, gastroparesis detected by solid-phase gastric emptying tests)

Functional dyspepsia: ulcer-like and dysmotility-like

Symptoms for which mechanisms have been proposed but as yet are poorly understood and for which confirmatory investigations are now being introduced. Probable mechanisms include:

- delayed gastric emptying
- uncoordinated relaxation of the gastric fundus
- hypersensitivity to gastric distension
- gastric dysrhythmias

Non-ulcer dyspepsia

- In the past this has meant ulcer-like symptoms in the absence of proven ulcer. It is a confusing term and ideally should be discarded.

in 1993. In the same year, over £400 million was spent on ulcer-healing drugs. In addition, sales of over-the-counter antacids accounted for £65 million. Worldwide expenditure on ulcer drugs for 1998 was approximately 11 billion US$; 4 billion US$ were spent on proton-pump inhibitors alone, of which nearly 50% were consumed in the USA.

Indirect costs and social consequences of dyspepsia are more difficult to measure. A UK survey in 1994 revealed that 40% of those with gastroesophageal reflux, 46% of gastric ulcer sufferers and 59% of duodenal ulcer patients had lost time from work in the previous 12 months because of their disease. By contrast there is evidence that appropriate treatment results in a lower rate of consultation and reduced healthcare costs.

Fast Facts – Dyspepsia provides an up-to-date account of our understanding of the main causes of dyspepsia and their management in the context of general practice.

Key references

Enck P, Dubois D, Maquis P. Quality of life in patients with upper gastrointestinal symptoms: results from the Domestic/International Gastroenterology Surveillance Study (DIGEST). *Scand J Gastroenterol* 1999;34(suppl 231):48–54.

Lydeard S, Jones R. Factors affecting the decision to consult with dyspepsia: a comparison of consulters with non-consulters. *J R Coll Gen Pract* 1989;39:495–8.

Meineche-Schmidt V, Talley NJ, Pap A et al. Impact of functional dyspepsia on quality of life and health care consumption after cessation of antisecretory treatment. *Scand J Gastroenterol* 1999;34:566–74.

Talley NJ, Zinmeister AR, Schleck CD, Melton III LJ. Dyspepsia and dyspepsia subgroups: a population based study. *Gastroenterology* 1992;102:1259–68.

1 Approaching uninvestigated dyspepsia

Patients with dyspepsia are not a homogeneous group, and their management therefore depends upon selection and prioritization.

Patients not requiring immediate investigation

Patients under the age of 45 years with a short history of dyspepsia may be treated empirically for 4–6 weeks, in the absence of alarm symptoms (Table 1.1). This approach prevents unnecessary investigation of many young patients with so-called 'self-limiting' dyspepsia and supposedly reduces management costs and inconvenience. Such a policy is valid provided:

- a significant proportion of young dyspeptics fall into this category
- the majority do not return because symptoms resolve or are subsequently controlled by over-the-counter drugs and lifestyle changes.

The overall success of this approach depends on:

- appropriate selection of patients
- the physician's clinical diagnostic skills
- the physician's ability to reassure and convince the patient that immediate investigation is unnecessary.

If not applied appropriately, however, the 'treat-before-investigation' approach may delay optimal management and prove less cost-effective. Doubts about this empirical approach have been strengthened by a study that randomized uninvestigated dyspeptics to early endoscopy or H_2-receptor antagonists therapy without investigation. At 12 months,

TABLE 1.1

Alarm symptoms

- Anemia
- Dysphagia
- Weight loss / anorexia
- Bleeding
- Persistent vomiting

costs were greater and satisfaction was lower in the empirically treated group. Furthermore the majority of the latter patients eventually underwent endoscopy because of recurrent symptoms.

Symptom clusters. In the recent past it was proposed that clusters of symptoms might be used as a guide to initial therapy of dyspepsia in young, uninvestigated patients (Table 1.2). This approach to early management was advocated on the assumption that, in each of these categories, the implied pathogenesis was operative in a substantial number of patients and that drug therapy selected on this basis had a reasonable chance of being effective. However, initial enthusiasm has been dampened by more critical studies. These have shown that there is substantial overlap between the cluster subgroups, poor correlation with subsequent investigation findings and ineffectiveness of therapy based on the implied diagnosis.

It is now accepted that heartburn is an accurate indication of gastroesophageal reflux, which may be appropriately confirmed by

TABLE 1.2

Symptom clusters in uninvestigated dyspepsia and gastroesophageal reflux disease

Gastroesophageal reflux disease-like

- Heartburn
- Regurgitation

Ulcer-like

- Localized epigastric pain
- Nocturnal pain
- Relief with antacids or vomiting

Dysmotility-like

- Poorly localized upper abdominal discomfort
- Early satiety
- Bloating
- Nausea

TABLE 1.3
Initial therapy according to predominant symptom

Dyspepsia type	Predominant symptom	Initial therapy
Ulcer-like	Epigastric pain	Acid suppression
Dysmotility-like	Upper abdominal discomfort	Prokinetic drug
Non-specific	Neither of the above predominate	

a beneficial response to 4 weeks of proton-pump inhibitor treatment. Such patients are now suitably excluded from the classification of uninvestigated dyspepsia.

Although diagnosis based on symptom clusters is no longer favoured, it has been proposed that the predominant symptom may be of value in predicting possible pathogenic mechanisms and, by implication, appropriate initial therapy (Table 1.3). Those with ulcer-like dyspepsia tend to be men with normal gastric emptying, while those with dysmotility-like symptoms are more often women with delayed gastric emptying and crossover symptoms with the irritable bowel syndrome.

***Helicobacter pylori* serological screening.** Because of the close association between *H. pylori* and organic causes of dyspepsia, serological screening has been used to guide initial management of young patients. One proposal is that *H. pylori*-positive patients should be referred for endoscopy and given eradication treatment if ulcer disease is confirmed. In the UK, this approach is probably not appropriate in general practice and is not cost-effective.

The alternative policy is to give eradication therapy to all young *H. pylori*-positive dyspeptics without alarm symptoms (Table 1.1, Figure 1.1). The rationale is that 20% will have ulcers, many others will have responsive mucosal lesions and, for the remainder, there is the potential to reduce the risk of future disease. This approach is advocated by the European *H. pylori* Study Group, the European Society for Primary Care Gastroenterology and the American Gastroenterological Association. However, many gastroenterologists in

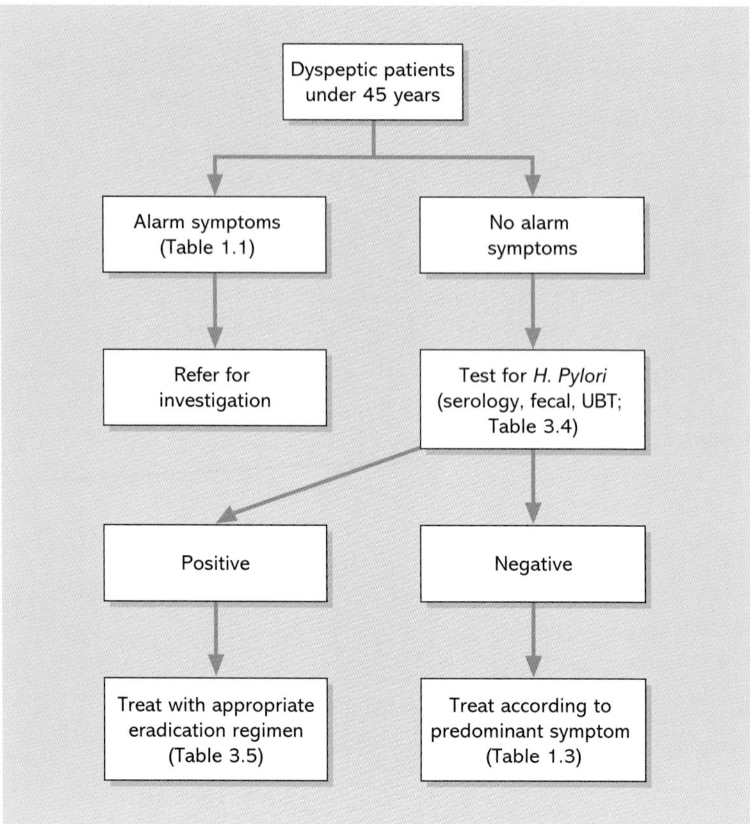

Figure 1.1 'Test and treat' guidelines for young patients. UBT, urea breath test.

secondary care reserve eradication therapy for patients with documented ulcer disease who test positive for *H. pylori*.

H. pylori-negative patients in this age group are unlikely to have major organic disease. Therefore, they may be treated according to their predominant symptom (Table 1.3) and only referred if unresponsive.

Patients requiring early investigation or referral

Patients with alarm features. Regardless of their age, all patients who have one or more alarm symptoms (Table 1.1) should be investigated promptly. These symptoms are frequently associated with serious organic disease.

Approaching uninvestigated dyspepsia – Key points

- Patients under 45 without alarm symptoms
  – treat empirically for 4–6 weeks
- Young *H. pylori*-positive patients
  – give eradication therapy
- Patients with alarm symptoms and those over 45
  – refer for investigation.

Patients over 45 years of age. The risk of organic disease increases with age. Any patient over 45 with recent onset of dyspepsia should be referred or investigated without delay, regardless of *H. pylori* status.

Patients with chronic symptoms. Many previously uninvestigated patients with significant long-standing dyspeptic symptoms or heartburn will have chronic organic disease. Those who have used antacids in large quantities on an almost daily basis for several years are particularly likely to have peptic disease. They need to be distinguished from those with non-acid-related functional dyspepsia to optimize future management.

Anxious or phobic patients. Some patients or their relatives will be dissatisfied with a symptom-based diagnosis. Early referral should then be conceded to facilitate future management. These patients include those with:

- excessive anxiety
- cancer phobia
- a vulnerable psychosocial background
- an associate with a recent history of serious disease.

Initial investigations for dyspepsia and esophageal symptoms

Upper gastrointestinal endoscopy is undoubtedly the most appropriate initial investigation, because of its capacity to confirm or exclude the majority of diseases that commonly cause dyspepsia (Table 1.4). The

TABLE 1.4

Endoscopy can identify conditions often associated with dyspepsia*

Finding	Patients (%)
Normal	38.0
Peptic ulcer	18.0
Esophagitis	15.0
Gastritis	18.0
Duodenitis	8.0
Carcinoma	1.8
Miscellaneous	1.2

*Data from Jones 1989

procedure is highly cost-effective because it often reduces the need for subsequent consultations and helps the physician to optimize drug therapy. As a result, most gastroenterologists strongly believe that patients with persistent or recurrent dyspepsia should undergo this investigation.

Upper gastrointestinal barium studies remain a valuable alternative to endoscopy for the confirmation or exclusion of peptic ulcer, esophageal strictures and neoplasia.

Abdominal ultrasound scanning has very limited value in the routine investigation of dyspepsia and should be reserved for patients with suspected biliary colic, cholecystitis, bile-duct obstruction or pancreatic disease. Note that vague pain in the right hypochondrium together with flatulence, once thought to be symptoms of cholelithiasis, are no more common in patients with gallstones than in those without.

Biochemical tests. Confirmed anemia increases the suspicion that dyspepsia has an organic cause. Abnormal liver biochemistry is found in some patients with biliary tract and pancreatic disease. However, the majority of dyspeptic patients have normal blood tests.

Key references

British Society of Gastroenterology Dyspepsia Management Guidelines. London, September 1996.

Bytzer P, Hansen J, Schaffalitzky de Muckadell OB. Empirical H_2 blocker therapy or prompt endoscopy in management of dyspepsia. *Lancet* 1994;343:811–16.

Bytzer P, Muller Hansen J, Schaffalitzky de Muckadell OB, Malchow-Moller A. Predicting endoscopic diagnosis in the dyspeptic patient. *Scand J Gastroenterol* 1997;32:118–25.

Delaney BC, Wilson S, Rolfe A et al. Randomised controlled trial of *H. pylori* testing and endoscopy for dyspepsia in primary care. *BMJ* 2001;322:898–901.

Jones C. *Practical Approach to Dyspepsia*. Oxford: The Medicine Group, 1989.

Lydeard S, Jones R. Factors affecting the decision to consult with dyspepsia: a comparison of consulters with non-consulters. *J R Coll Gen Pract* 1989;39:495–8.

Talley NJ, Stanghellini V, Heading RC et al. Functional gastroduodenal disorders. *Gut* 1999;45(suppl 2): II37–42.

Talley NJ, Zimsmeister AR, Schleck CD, Melthon III LJ. Dyspepsia and dyspepsia subgroups: a population study. *Gastroenterology* 1992;102:1259–68.

2 Gastroesophageal reflux disease

Symptoms of gastroesophageal reflux disease (GERD) often result from disordered esophagogastric motility, which facilitates the escape of normally secreted gastric acid into the distal esophagus for an abnormally long time.

Pathophysiology

The pathophysiology of GERD encompasses a continuum ranging from:

- reflux of small amounts of acid with persistent symptoms, to
- severe ulceration with stricture formation and dysphagia, to
- an inflammatory alteration of mucosal epithelium, to
- intestinal dysplasia, cellular atypia and adenocarcinoma.

Small amounts of acid reflux from the stomach into the esophagus occur on a daily basis in healthy individuals. Studies indicate that, for 1–6% of a 24-hour day, pH in the distal esophagus transiently falls below 4. So, for most of the time, acid in the stomach lumen is retained in the stomach.

Normal neuromuscular activities of the esophagus and stomach (esophagogastric motility) ensure that acid remains in the stomach or is emptied into the duodenum, and that very little refluxes into the esophagus. These activities include:

- normal esophageal peristalsis
- normal lower esophageal sphincter (LES) pressure
- a normal number of transient LES relaxations
- normal gastric emptying.

Disorders of esophageal and gastric motility associated with acidic reflux are listed in Table 2.1. Other esophageal defenses are the cardiac glands within the distal esophageal squamous epithelium, which secrete bicarbonate, and normal secretion of saliva, which is rich in bicarbonate.

Hypersecretory states present an additional challenge for the neuromuscular and epithelial defences of the esophagus. In Zollinger–

TABLE 2.1

Pathogenesis of GERD

Dysmotility	Toxic refluxates
• Failed esophageal peristalsis • Decreased amplitude of esophageal contractions • Hypotensive LES • Transient relaxation of LES pressure	• Gastric acid • Pepsin • Bile

LES, lower esophageal sphincter

Ellison syndrome, gastric and duodenal ulcerations are the major problems, but 40–60% of patients also have reflux esophagitis. The majority of patients with GERD, however, have normal acid secretory status and only a minority have idiopathic acid hypersecretion.

Dysfunction of the esophageal body. Studies from otherwise healthy individuals with GERD have shown that increasing mucosal damage (i.e. from mild to severe esophagitis) is associated with increasing contractile abnormalities of the esophageal body. Healthy control subjects fail to elicit a normal esophageal peristaltic wave after 10% of voluntary swallows, but patients with severe esophagitis fail to have normal peristaltic contractions after 30% of voluntary swallows. Thus, swallowed saliva often fails to reach the distal portions of the esophagus and to neutralize refluxed acid (Figure 2.1).

The amplitude of esophageal contractions may also be decreased in patients with reflux esophagitis. Even when acute inflammation is healed, neither the amplitude of contractions nor the frequency of normal esophageal peristalsis improves. Thus, the patient with GERD and esophagitis has fixed underlying esophageal motility abnormalities.

Dysfunction of the lower esophageal sphincter. Lower-esophageal sphincter pressure was at one time believed to be the chief defense against GERD (Figure 2.1). Numerous studies showed that patients with severe erosive esophagitis and regurgitation often had LES pressures below 10 mmHg (normal LES pressure is 12–40 mmHg). When LES pressure is below 10 mmHg, small increases in intra-abdominal pressure (such as those that occur when bending over or after eating a large meal) often result in free reflux of gastric contents into the esophagus.

However, many patients with severe heartburn have entirely normal resting LES pressures. The most common mechanism by which acid refluxes from the stomach into the esophagus is related to transient and inappropriate LES relaxations (Figure 2.2). In these instances, the normal resting LES pressure spontaneously reduces. This transient relaxation presents an opportunity for acid reflux to occur. In mild GERD, there is an increased number of transient LES relaxations; as the number of transient relaxations increases, the severity of esophagitis increases.

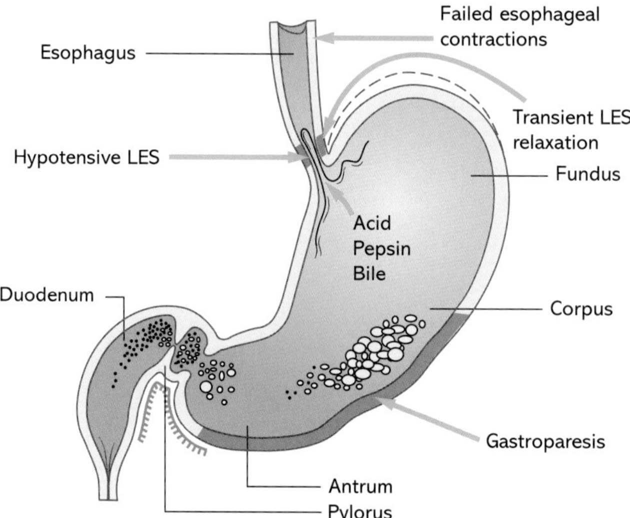

Figure 2.1 Pathophysiology of GERD includes esophageal and gastric motility disturbances related to failed esophageal peristalsis, hypotensive lower esophageal sphincter (LES), transient and inappropriate relaxation of the LES, and gastric dysmotility (gastroparesis). Dysmotility allows the reflux of toxic substances (acid, pepsin or bile) into the esophagus.

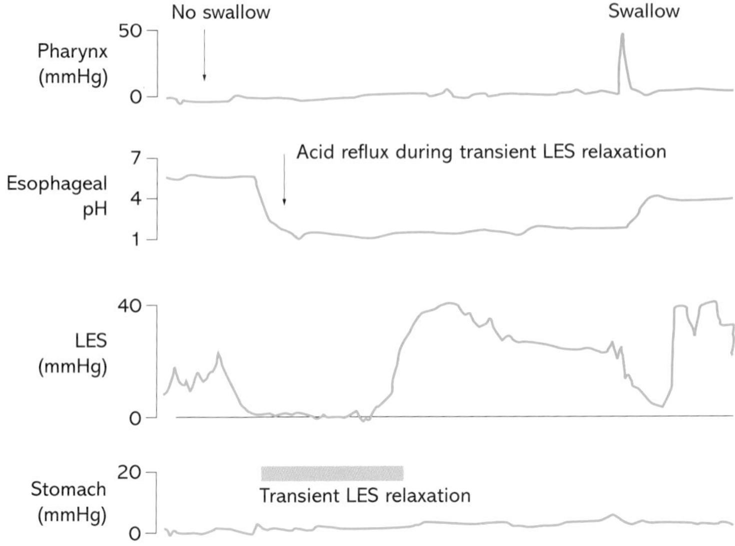

Figure 2.2 Transient LES relaxation and GERD. In the absence of a swallow, the LES relaxes to intragastric pressure for a prolonged period of time. After several seconds of transient LES relaxation, acid reflux occurs as indicated by the decrease in esophageal pH from 6 to 1. Reproduced with permission from Holloway RH. *Am J Physiol* 1995;268:G128–33.

Gastric dysmotility. Gastric emptying of chyme occurs, almost linearly, over 90–120 minutes after ingestion of solid foods. Abnormalities in gastric emptying have been recorded in 30–40% of patients with GERD. In some, emptying of standard meals (usually technetium-labeled eggs or liver) is significantly delayed (gastroparesis) compared with control subjects. As gastric acid and chyme remain in the stomach for longer times if gastroparesis is present, the risk of reflux is increased, particularly when LES pressure is very low and during transient esophageal sphincter relaxations.

Gastric acid, bile and pancreatic juices. The most injurious agent in GERD appears to be gastric acid. Most patients with GERD, however, have normal acid secretion. Therefore, normal amounts of acid can cause symptoms and mucosal damage if the esophageal epithelium is in contact with acid for prolonged periods of time. A small percentage of patients with GERD also reflux bile, with or without acid, into the esophagus. Pancreatic juices may also be toxic to the squamous epithelium of the distal esophagus; very little is known about this mechanism of injury.

Causes of neuromuscular damage to the esophagus and stomach in most patients with GERD are unknown. However, certain systemic disorders may affect esophageal neuromuscular function and increase the risk of gastroesophageal reflux. With scleroderma, for example, type I collagen is deposited in the submucosal tissues. Eventually, enteric neurons are destroyed and normal smooth muscle cells are replaced with collagen, resulting in decreased esophageal muscle function. Thus, the amplitude of peristaltic contractions decreases until eventually few or no contractions occur in the rigid sclerodermatous esophageal body. Similarly, LES pressure decreases markedly in scleroderma as sphincter muscles are weakened and replaced by collagen deposits, and free reflux occurs. Patients with scleroderma and the CRST syndrome (calcinosis, Raynaud's phenomenon, sclerodactyly and telangiectasia), in particular, are at high risk for esophagitis and esophagitis-related peptic strictures.

Chronic sequelae. Many patients with chronic reflux and classic heartburn symptoms will have virtually no observable damage in the esophageal mucosa at endoscopy. Increased eosinophilia and acute inflammatory cells may be seen in histological sections of biopsies from apparently normal distal esophagus. On the other hand, recurrent acid reflux may lead to obvious esophageal ulcers.

Esophagitis is graded from 1 (mild) to 3 (erosive). The intermittent inflammation and healing process may lead to peptic strictures in the distal esophagus in some patients. Other patients with chronic GERD may develop Barrett's epithelium, which may range from the gastric to the intestinal type. The intestinal type is more likely to develop areas of dysplasia, cellular atypia and adenocarcinoma. Severe atypia is associated with a high risk of adenocarcinoma of the esophagus.

Symptoms

Diagnosis is based on clinical symptoms, the most common being heartburn (Table 2.2). Atypical GERD symptoms caused by acid reflux into the esophagus, pharynx, lungs and throat constitute another important clinical area for consideration. Typical or atypical angina-like chest discomfort, nausea, nocturnal asthma attacks, aspiration pneumonia, chronic hoarseness and a variety of other symptoms may be related to gastroesophageal reflux.

Heartburn is the most common symptom associated with GERD. It is defined as a burning sensation high in the epigastrium that *rises* into the subxiphoid or substernal areas. Burning may be felt higher in the retrosternal region and into the back of the throat. Heartburn may be accompanied by increased salivation or pressure discomfort in the retrosternal area. It typically occurs in the postprandial hours and may

TABLE 2.2

Clinical symptoms of GERD

Symptom	Noted by
Typical	
• Heartburn	
• Regurgitation	
• Belching	
Atypical	
• Halitosis • Dental erosions	May be noted by dentist
• Hoarseness • Chronic cough	May be noted by otolaryngologist
• Episodic asthma	May be noted by chest physician
• Substernal discomfort, angina pectoris	May be noted by cardiologist
• Nausea • Early satiety, fullness, bloating (associated with gastric dysmotility)	May be noted by gastroenterologist

also occur at night when the patient is supine. Nocturnal heartburn is associated with increased severity of esophagitis and stricture formation.

In most people, heartburn is transient and related to over-indulgence in a wide variety of rich or acidic foods. Over-the-counter antacids have traditionally been the treatment of choice for simple heartburn. The recently available over-the-counter H_2-receptor antagonists have given individuals access to systemic medications to decrease gastric acid secretion and reduce self-diagnosed heartburn symptoms. However, millions of patients have persistent and chronic heartburn symptoms that are troublesome and may also lead to serious sequelae, such as:

- gastrointestinal bleeding from esophageal erosions and ulcers
- peptic stricture formation
- formation of Barrett's epithelium, with an attendant increase in the incidence of adenocarcinoma of the esophagus.

Alarm symptoms. If a patient over 50 years of age has heartburn and one or more alarm symptoms (Table 2.3), heartburn should be addressed with more aggressive diagnostic and therapeutic action.

Dysphagia for solids, but not liquids, may indicate mechanical obstruction of the esophagus. The key possibilities include:

- peptic stricture
- esophageal rings or webs
- distal esophageal squamous cell carcinoma or adenocarcinoma.

Odynophagia (pain on swallowing, rather than a burning sensation rising into the retrosternal area) suggests an infectious esophagitis

TABLE 2.3

Alarm symptoms

- Dysphagia
- Odynophagia
- Weight loss
- Blood in regurgitant fluids or vomitus

caused by *Candida* or herpes simplex virus. Immunocompromised patients may have one of these atypical causes of their heartburn or odynophagia. Weight loss, melena or anemia suggest the possibility of esophageal or gastric cancer. Scleroderma and pill-induced esophagitis should be considered. Potassium tablets, salicylates and alendronate sodium are frequent causes of pill-induced esophagitis.

Atypical symptoms. Over the past several years, interest in atypical presentations of GERD (see Table 2.2) has increased in medical and surgical specialties ranging from dentistry to cardiology. Atypical symptoms that may present in the dental realm include loss of dental enamel and halitosis. Ear, nose and throat physicians have determined that patients with chronic hoarseness and sore throat frequently have occult GERD. Many of these patients do not report heartburn symptoms. If present, they may be unimportant to the patient compared with the throat symptoms.

Pulmonary physicians appreciate that gastroesophageal reflux is frequently present in asthmatic patients. Nocturnal asthma attacks or microaspiration may be precipitated by GERD. Similarly, chronic cough is stimulated by gastroesophageal reflux in some patients. In a recent study, patients with severe chronic obstructive pulmonary or bronchospastic disease underwent Nissen fundoplication (see pages 29–30); the incidence of reflux and severity of pulmonary symptoms decreased significantly as a result.

In other patients, reflux of acid into the esophagus is perceived as a pressure discomfort or heaviness rather than a burning sensation. Some patients may have no burning at all and acid reflux is experienced as a squeezing pressure or substernal pain that suggests angina pectoris. Reflux of acid into the esophagus probably causes an angina-like pain by either:

- stimulating a sensory reflex
- inducing focal ischemia in the esophageal muscular wall
- stimulating esophageal smooth muscle spasm.

Other gastrointestinal symptoms may be associated with GERD. In a series of patients with chronic unexplained nausea, occult GERD was present and episodes of nausea were associated with acid reflux recorded during 24-hour esophageal pH studies. Aggressive anti-secretory and promotility therapy improved the nausea.

Many patients with heartburn also have symptoms associated with gastric emptying disorders, such as excess postprandial fullness, early satiety, nausea, vomiting and epigastric discomfort. These patients have an overlap syndrome in which GERD and symptoms associated with dysmotility-like dyspepsia are present.

Finally, patients with Barrett's epithelium may have very minor heartburn symptoms. As the squamous mucosa changes to the gastric or intestinal type, it becomes less sensitive to acid exposure from a symptomatic viewpoint. In patients who have had mild reflux for many years, the possibility of Barrett's epithelium should be considered.

Diagnosis

The basic approach to the management of GERD is to make the clinical diagnosis in patients with classical symptoms and to be suspicious of GERD in patients with atypical symptoms. In the patient with classical symptoms of GERD, it is important to consider underlying systemic disorders that might be causing the symptoms and to check for the presence of alarm symptoms as described previously. The presence of dysphagia and the chronicity of relatively mild heartburn should also raise concerns regarding Barrett's epithelium and the complications thereof. Dysphagia, odynophagia or other alarm symptoms indicate that a more aggressive and definitive diagnostic approach should be taken.

Barium-swallow examination is the minimum esophageal evaluation required for patients with one or more alarm symptoms. Barium-swallow radiographs will show large ulcers, masses and other structural defects that may be causing the symptoms. Structural defects detected on barium swallow must be evaluated with UGI endoscopy and be biopsied for malignancy if suspicious. Depending on the services available, UGI endoscopy should be the initial diagnostic procedure of choice in the presence of alarm symptoms.

Endoscopy. As the intensity of heartburn symptoms does not correlate well with endoscopic findings, it is helpful to use endoscopy for those patients who have classical GERD symptoms but are not responding to standard treatment approaches (see page 26). Upper endoscopic examination may reveal an entirely normal esophageal mucosa or a continuum of endoscopic findings, from streaky erythematous areas to obvious ulcerations of the squamous epithelium. Peptic or cancerous strictures or Barrett's epithelium may be detected. Retained food in the stomach suggests neuromuscular abnormalities of the stomach, and large amounts of bile suggest duodenogastric reflux. A solid-phase gastric-emptying study will confirm the diagnosis of gastroparesis. Electrogastrography will indicate the presence of gastric dysrhythmia which occurs in almost 80% of patients with heartburn *and* dysmotility-like dyspepsia symptoms (GERD plus). These two non-invasive tests of gastric motility are described further in Chapter 6.

Other tests. If barium-swallow or endoscopic studies of the esophagus, stomach and duodenum are entirely normal and the patient continues to have heartburn despite standard therapies, determination of esophageal motility and 24-hour pH measurements may be needed. Esophageal manometry will detect a hypotensive LES and indicate the continuing high risk for recurrent reflux or regurgitation. On the other hand, the LES pressure may be normal, which suggests that the main mechanism of reflux is transient relaxation of the sphincter. Other unsuspected esophageal motility disorders may be found, such as achalasia or findings suggestive of scleroderma. A 24-hour esophageal pH study will determine the extent to which the esophageal mucosa is exposed to gastric acid. The patient records all heartburn episodes and the time of symptoms in a diary, so that the physician can correlate reflux events with the occurrence of symptoms. GERD may not, in fact, be documented. A positive result may confirm the diagnosis of GERD as a cause of atypical symptoms.

Atypical GERD symptoms, such as chronic cough, hoarseness, episodic asthma and angina-like chest discomfort require a confirmatory 24-hour esophageal pH study. The time of symptom occurrence and the correlation between symptoms and individual reflux events should be documented carefully.

Treatment

Treatment of GERD is organized into a series of stages.

- Stage I involves lifestyle and behavior modifications.
- Stage II consists of treatment with systemic drugs, such as H_2-receptor antagonists, prokinetic agents and proton-pump inhibitors.
- Stage III includes surgical procedures, such as Nissen fundoplication, or endoscopic procedures such as radiofrequency ablation or endoluminal plication techniques.

Stage I. During this stage, the physician seeks to identify risk factors in the patient's lifestyle that might contribute to GERD symptoms. Certain foods, particularly citric juices, and tomato- and onion-based spices or foods, are commonly associated with increased heartburn symptoms. Chocolate, alcohol and nicotine decrease LES pressure to some degree and increase the likelihood of reflux symptoms. Other lifestyle changes include decreasing the volume of food ingested at the evening meal and eating at an earlier time to avoid sleeping with a full stomach. The head of the patient's bed may be placed on 4–6-inch (10–15-cm) blocks so that gravity helps to prevent stomach contents from refluxing into the esophagus.

The physician should also review the patient's medications to identify those drugs that decrease LES pressure (calcium-channel blockers and drugs containing theophylline) or decrease gastric emptying rates (anticholinergic drugs and opioids). If possible, these drugs should be stopped to see if symptoms improve.

Most patients will have tried over-the-counter antacids. The availability of over-the-counter H_2-receptor antagonists has increased the likelihood that the patient will have tried these drugs; if they do not relieve the symptoms of GERD, patients are often motivated to seek medical attention. Physicians who diagnose GERD typically prescribe H_2-receptor antagonists at higher doses than are available over the counter. When stage I approaches fail to relieve symptoms, stage II therapies should be considered.

Stage II. In the presence of classical heartburn symptoms, the physician can address either the acid secretion or the relevant esophagogastric dysmotility aspects of GERD.

H_2-receptor antagonists include cimetidine, ranitidine, nizatidine and famotidine (Table 2.4). They differ in potency, but overall effectiveness is approximately the same. H_2-receptor antagonists heal endoscopically proven esophagitis in about 50% of patients at 8 weeks and up to 70% at 12 weeks.

Proton-pump inhibitors (PPIs), such as omeprazole, lansoprazole, pantoprazole and rabeprazole, are the most potent acid-inhibiting agents available. Acid inhibition is significantly greater with this type

TABLE 2.4

Medical treatments for GERD

Class and drug	Dose	Endoscopic improvement (%)*
H_2-receptor antagonist		
Cimetidine	400 mg, four times a day	~70
Ranitidine	150–300 mg,** twice a day	~80
Famotidine	20–40 mg, twice a day	~80
Nizatidine	150 mg, twice a day	~50
Proton-pump inhibitors		
Omeprazole	20–40 mg, once a day	~90
Lansoprazole	30 mg, once a day	~90
Rabeprazole	20 mg, once a day	~90
Pantoprazole	40 mg, once a day	~90
Esomeprazole	20 mg, once a day	~90
Prokinetic agents		
Metoclopramide	10 mg, four times a day	~70

*Data from Bell and Hunt 1991

**The higher dose may be needed if the patient has erosive changes or is symptomatically resistant to the lower dose of drug than with the H_2-receptor antagonists. Recommended doses to achieve greater than 90% healing rates for endoscopically proven esophagitis are 20 mg once a day for omeprazole, or 30 mg once a day for lansoprazole, or 40 mg once a day for pantoprazole, or 20 mg once a day for rabeprazole, for routine purposes. For resistant cases, 20 mg twice a day, or 40 mg once a day, of omeprazole should be given. Proton-pump inhibitors are very effective for healing severe, erosive esophagitis. Whether they should be first-line treatment for patients with heartburn or used after H_2-receptor antagonists or prokinetic agents have failed to relieve symptoms adequately remains controversial. Long-term use of omeprazole is associated with elevated gastrin levels and chronic atrophic gastritis, but gastric carcinoids or other serious sequelae have not been reported.

Carafate, available in the USA, is a complex carbohydrate in oral suspension that can also be used to provide topical healing for esophagitis and heartburn.

Metoclopramide is a centrally and peripherally acting dopamine-2 (D_2) antagonist that increases the LES pressure and the rate of gastric emptying. It can be given orally or by intravenous infusion. The usual dose is 10 mg three or four times a day in the UK. In the USA, the usual dose is 10–15 mg four times a day. However, approximately 20–30% of patients will experience side-effects related to central nervous system events, including depression, anxiety and tardive dyskinesia.

Domperidone is a drug with a similar pharmacological action to that of metoclopramide, but with a lower side-effect profile. It is available in Europe, but not in the USA.

Cisapride was approved in the USA for the treatment of nocturnal heartburn, but has been withdrawn from the market. Cisapride is associated with an increase in the risk for QT prolongation, torsade de pointes and ventricular dysrhythmia, particularly in patients with heart disease. Also, drugs that increase cisapride blood levels by interfering with cisapride metabolism at the hepatic cytochrome P450 3A4 carry a small, but increased, risk of significant cardiac dysrhythmia. As a result, cisapride is contraindicated in combination with erythromycin and other macrolides, antifungal agents, protease inhibitors and the antidepressant drug paroxetine.

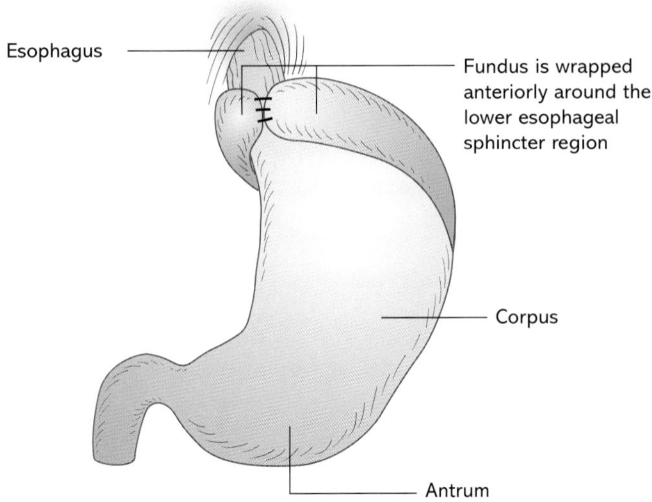

Figure 2.3 The Nissen fundoplication operation for drug-refractory GERD symptoms.

Stage III. Younger patients requiring high doses of expensive medications to control GERD symptoms may be candidates for surgery.

The Nissen fundoplication operation is the most commonly performed surgical procedure for GERD. The procedure provides relief from GERD symptoms for about 10 years. The gastric fundus is wrapped around itself and the distal esophagus, and any hiatal hernia is reduced (Figure 2.3). When the operation is successful, over 85% of patients will have no heartburn or regurgitation and medications for GERD symptoms may be reduced or stopped. The procedure decreases the incidence of transient lower esophageal relaxations and increases LES pressure. After Nissen fundoplication, a minority of patients may have difficulty with swallowing and/or belching and may suffer 'gas bloat'.

Nissen fundoplication should not be performed until an esophageal manometry study has shown low or low–normal LES pressure. In addition, achalasia, diffuse esophageal spasm or severe non-specific contractile abnormalities of the esophageal body should be excluded before this surgery. Patients with scleroderma and GERD symptoms should not have a Nissen fundoplication, because dysphagia is increased.

If symptoms suggestive of dysmotility-like dyspepsia are present, an electrogastrogram test and a gastric emptying study should be considered before surgery. The effect of fundoplication on existing gastroparesis may improve emptying in some patients, but gastroparesis has also been reported after fundoplication. Nissen fundoplication can be performed laparoscopically, and results appear to be satisfactory and comparable to the open approach when carried out by experienced surgeons.

Two endoscopic procedures for the treatment of GERD were recently approved by the Food and Drug Administration (FDA) in the USA. Radiofrequency therapy applied to the LES and cardia region has been found to decrease transient LES relaxation and to be associated with improved heartburn symptoms. A diagram of the procedure is shown in Figure 2.4. The technique reduces transient lower esophageal sphincter relaxation. Long-term trials and results over 2 years are positive. Another endoscopic technique uses a sewing-machine-like device to plicate a fold of fundic mucosa near the cardia. Long-term trials and results have not been published.

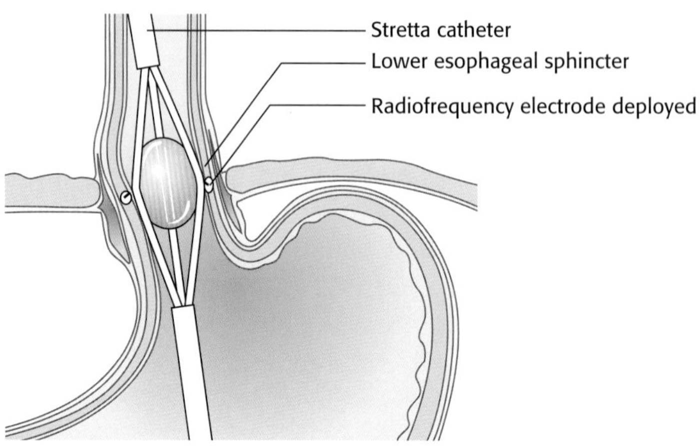

Figure 2.4 Radiofrequency therapy applied to LES and cardia.

Gastroesophageal reflux disease – Key points

- Transient lower esophageal sphincter relaxation and poor acid clearance from the esophageal body are the key pathophysiological events in GERD.
- PPIs and H_2-receptor blocking agents are safe and effective inhibitors of acid secretion for treatment of heartburn.
- Barrett's epithelium and adenocarcinoma of the esophagus are sequelae of longstanding gastroesophageal reflux.
- Nissen fundoplication remains the antireflux operation of choice, but the role of endoscopic techniques in GERD therapy is evolving.

Key references

Barlow AB, DeMeester TR, Ball CS et al. The significance of the gastric secretory state in gastroesophageal reflux disease. *Arch Surg* 1989;124:937–40.

Brzana RJ, Koch KL. Intractable nausea presenting as gastroesophageal reflux disease. *Ann Intern Med* 1997;126:704–7.

El-Searg HB, Sonnenberg A. Comorbid occurrence of laryngeal or pulmonary disease with esophagitis in United States' military veterans. *Gastroenterology* 1997;113:755–60.

Fennerty MB, Sampliner RE, Garewell HS. Review: Barrett's oesophagus – cancer risk, biology and therapeutic management. *Aliment Pharmacol Ther* 1993;7:339–45.

Hinder RA, Filipi CJ, Wetschler G et al. Laparoscopic Nissen fundoplication is an effective treatment for gastroesophageal reflux disease. *Ann Surg* 1994;220:472–83.

Katz PO. Pathogenesis and management of gastroesophageal reflux disease. *J Clin Gastroenterol* 1991;113:S6–15.

Klinkenberg-Knoll EC, Festen HPM, Jansen JBMJ et al. Long-term treatment with omeprazole for refractory reflux esophagitis: efficacy and safety. *Ann Intern Med* 1994;121:161–7.

Mittal R, McCallum RW. Characteristics and frequency of transient relaxations of the lower esophageal sphincter in patients with reflux esophagitis. *Gastroenterology* 1988;95:593–9.

Orlando RC. Reflux esophagitis. In: T Yamada, ed. *Textbook of Gastroenterology*. Philadelphia: JB Lippincott, 1995:1318–46.

Schnatz PF, Castell JA, Castell DO. Pulmonary symptoms associated with gastroesophageal reflux: use of ambulatory pH monitoring to diagnose and to direct therapy. *Am J Gastroenterol* 1996;91:1715–18.

Triadafilopoulis G, DiBaise JK, Nostrant TT et al. The Stretta procedure for the treatment of GERD: 6 and 12 month follow-up of the US open label trial. *Gastrointest Endosc* 2002;55:149–56.

Viaezi MF, Richter JE. Role of acid and duodenogastroesophageal reflux in gastroesophageal reflux disease. *Gastroenterology* 1996;111:1192–9.

Although spiral bacteria in the stomach have been reported by numerous observers since the 19th century, it was not until 1982 that Marshall and Warren cultured the organism that was later to be named *Helicobacter pylori* and which today is known to be prevalent worldwide (Figure 3.1). They and others rapidly recognized its close association with gastritis and peptic ulceration; more recently, its etiological importance in gastric carcinoma and B-cell mucosa-associated lymphoid tissue (MALT) lymphoma has been established (Figure 3.2). There can be few discoveries that have so dramatically changed our understanding and management of such universal diseases.

Bacteriological features

H. pylori is a spiral, flagellate, Gram-negative, micro-aerophilic bacterium. It is uniquely adapted to survive in the hostile environment

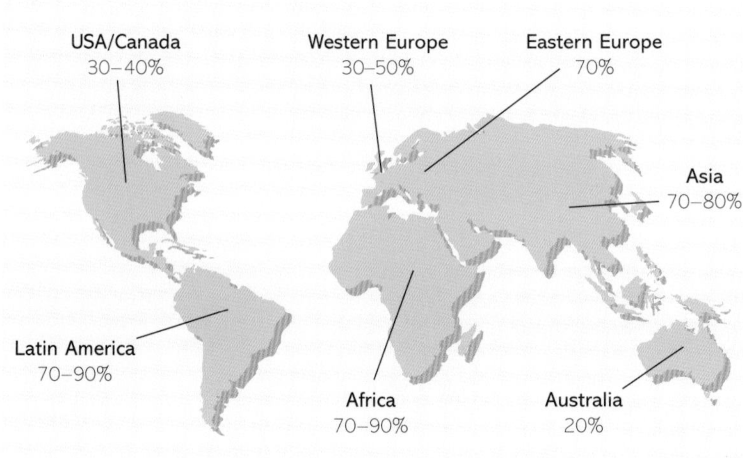

Figure 3.1 *H. pylori* is a ubiquitous organism with highest prevalence rates in the developing world. Reproduced with permission from Marshall BJ. *JAMA* 1995; 274:1064–6. © American Medical Association.

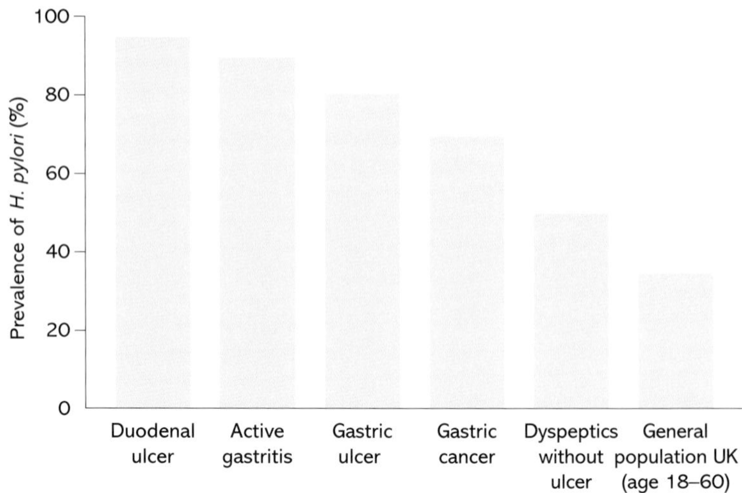

Figure 3.2 There is a strong association between peptic ulcer, gastritis, gastric malignancy and *H. pylori* infection.

of the stomach. The bacterium establishes itself by excluding acid from its immediate surroundings. It does so by converting naturally-occurring urea into carbon dioxide and ammonia, and expelling hydrogen ions using its own proton pump.

H. pylori is highly motile, so it is able to exist in both the gastric lumen and the mucus gel layer. It also possesses powerful adhesins, by which it attaches firmly to gastric epithelial cells where release of toxins initiates tissue damage and inflammation. It shows considerable diversity of toxin production, which probably explains why certain strains are more strongly associated with gastroduodenal diseases than others.

Infection: when, who and how

Age of infection. In the Western world, the prevalence of infection increases with age (Figure 3.3). However, it now seems that rather than being due to a steady acquisition of infection during adult life, this reflects a cohort effect. The elevated level of infection in those who are now elderly is the result of a high incidence of infection when they were young. Similarly, the lower prevalence in today's younger adults is the result of a falling incidence of infection during their childhood and

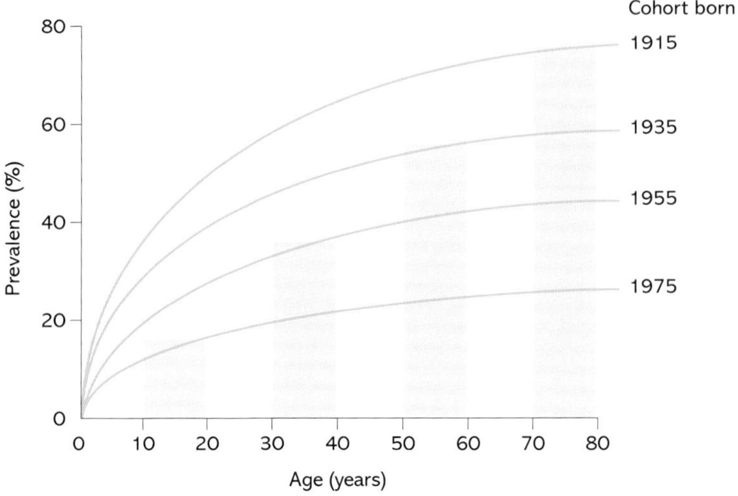

Figure 3.3 Birth cohort prevalence rates of *H. pylori* chronic infection (lines); prevalence of *H. pylori* according to age in the population today (bars) (from Sipponen P, Marshall BJ. *Gastroenterol Clin North Am* 2000;29:579–92).

adolescence, probably as a result of improved socioeconomic conditions. In contrast, the overwhelming majority of the population of developing countries continues to become infected before they are 20 years old (Figure 3.4). Regardless of geography, risk of acquisition is greatest during childhood, though up to 0.5% of adults in industrialized countries still become infected annually. Reinfection after eradication in developed countries is less than 1% per annum, but rates as high as 15% have been reported in the developing world.

Socioeconomic factors. In developed and developing countries, the prevalence of *H. pylori* infection is directly proportional to the level of socioeconomic deprivation, whether measured by education, income, occupation or living conditions. Children are most vulnerable and act as vectors of infection between adults.

Source and route of infection. It has been suggested that domestic and abattoir-slaughtered animals might act as a possible reservoir for

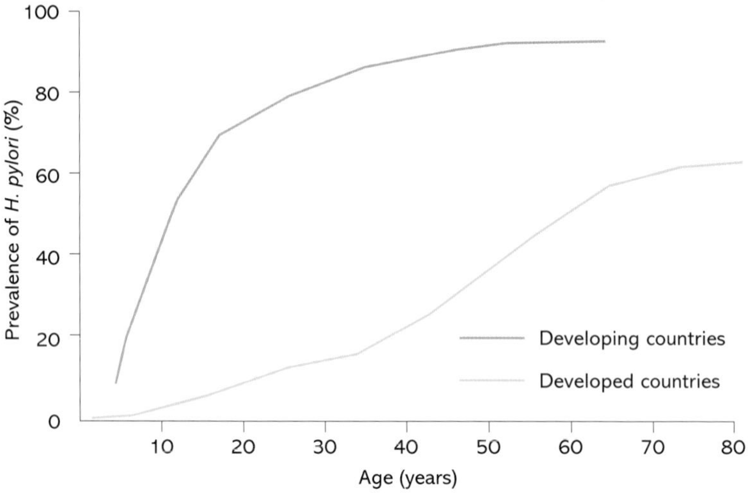

Figure 3.4 In the developed world, prevalence of *H. pylori* rises steadily with age, whereas the great majority of the population in developing countries is infected before the age of 20. Reproduced with permission from Northfield et al. *Helicobacter Pylori Infection*. Dordrecht: Kluwer, 1993. © 1993 Kluwer.

human infection. As for other gastrointestinal infections, drinking water in the developing world is also a potential source of infection. Direct, person-to-person spread is suggested by the increased prevalence of infection in residential institutions and families.

Isolation of *H. pylori* from dental plaque and vomit supports the contention that oral–oral transmission may occur. However, the organism retains viability in feces, and the fecal–oral route of infection is potentially more universal. Sources and routes of *H. pylori* infection are shown in Table 3.1.

Diseases associated with infection

Acute gastritis. Initial infection of the stomach may be asymptomatic, but some patients experience an illness lasting 1–2 weeks that includes epigastric pain, vomiting, nausea and occasionally pyrexia. This phase is accompanied by achlorhydria, which may take several months to resolve. Some patients spontaneously clear the organism, but the majority remain chronically infected.

TABLE 3.1

Possible sources and routes of transmission of *H. pylori*

Hosts	
• Primary	• Reservoir
– humans	– cats (proven)
	– pigs (suspected)
	– monkey (proven)
Routes and modes of contamination	
• Fecal–oral?	• Oral–oral
– uncooked vegetables	– vomitus
– surface (or well) water swimming/ingestion	– kissing

Chronic gastritis. The severity and distribution of chronic *H. pylori* infection is likely to depend upon bacterial characteristics, host response and environmental factors (Table 3.2). Interaction between these factors results in three distinct patterns of gastritis and subsequent morbidity (Figure 3.5).

Pan-gastritis patients have normal parietal cell mass but a premorbid reduced response to gastrin (Figure 3.5a). *H. pylori* is able to infect the body of the stomach as well as the antrum because, unlike in duodenal ulcer patients, there is no excess acid secretion from this part of the stomach. Despite elevated levels of serum gastrin following infection, excess acid secretion does not occur, because parietal cell function is impaired further by *H. pylori* infection of the gastric body. The great majority of these patients remain asymptomatic.

Antral gastritis. This is associated with duodenal ulcer (Figure 3.5b). *H. pylori* infection is restricted to the antrum in those patients with a premorbid, probably genetically determined, increased parietal cell mass in the corpus (where colonization is prevented by elevated acid secretion). Infection of the antrum leads to hypergastrinemia (see *Duodenal ulcer*, pages 52–54), which stimulates

TABLE 3.2

Factors that may influence the consequences of *H. pylori* infection

Bacterial characteristics

- Initial bacterial load
- Toxin production (cagA and vacA are associated with ulcer and gastric cancer)
- Adhesins

Host response

- HLA type and expression on gastric epithelium
- IgA response relative to IgM and IgG response
- Variable release of prostaglandins and leukotrienes
- Parietal cell mass and acid secretion
- Duodenogastric reflux
- Vascularity of gastric mucosa

Environmental factors

- Age at time of infection
- Dietary factors (excess salt and nitrates, vitamin C and E deficiencies)
- Non-steroidal anti-inflammatory drugs

HLA, human leukocyte antigen

the increased parietal cell mass to secrete excess acid that, in turn, induces gastric metaplasia in the duodenal mucosa, allowing *H. pylori* colonization.

Gastritis of the corpus. This is associated with gastric ulcer and adenocarcinoma (Figure 3.5c). Exposure to *H. pylori* in early childhood may predispose patients to infection of the gastric body with sparing of the antrum, resulting in atrophy of the parietal cell area, reduced acid secretion and secondary hypergastrinemia. Atrophy and achlorhydria might enhance ulcerogenic cofactors such as non-steroidal anti-inflammatory drugs (NSAIDs) and refluxed bile. Intestinal metaplasia accompanies severe and long-standing gastric atrophy, both of which are known predisposing factors

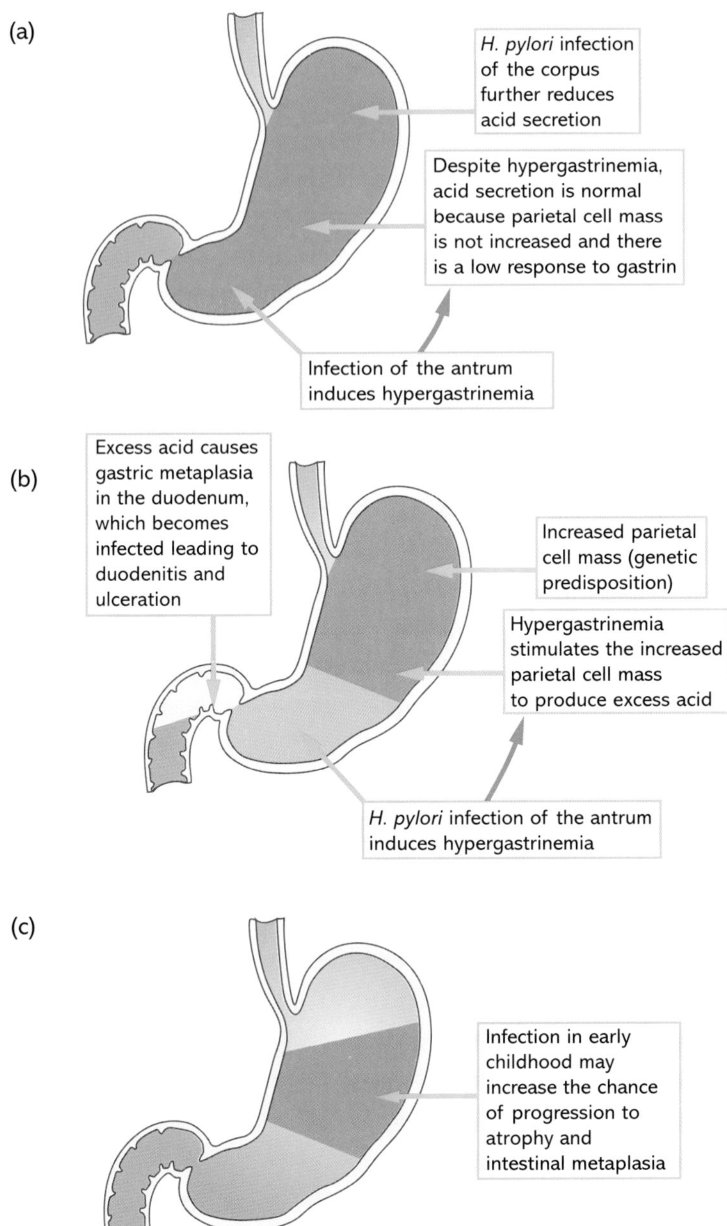

Figure 3.5 The three distinct patterns of gastritis: (a) pan-gastritis; (b) antral gastritis; and (c) gastritis of the corpus.

for carcinoma of the stomach. Achlorhydria encourages bacterial overgrowth, which enhances production of carcinogens.

Duodenal and gastric ulcer. The role of *H. pylori* in the pathogenesis of duodenal and gastric ulcer is described in Chapter 4.

Gastric cancer. Worldwide, gastric carcinoma is the second most common cancer, affecting up to 10 million people annually. *H. pylori* was designated a Class 1 carcinogen by the World Health Organization in 1994. Epidemiological evidence and the fact that *H. pylori* is accompanied by mucosal changes conducive to carcinogenesis support the association of *H. pylori* infection with gastric cancer (Table 3.3).

Potential for prevention. It seems likely that prevention or treatment of infection during childhood is likely to have the greatest impact on reducing the subsequent development of gastric cancer. The effect of improved living standards is already evident in industrialized countries. Childhood screening combined with eradication therapy may further reduce the risk, though this strategy has less potential in the developing world where reinfection rates are high. Whether eradication therapy in adults prevents progression of carcinogenesis remains to be proved. In worldwide terms, a significant

TABLE 3.3

Evidence to support an association between gastric cancer and *H. pylori*

- There is worldwide correlation between prevalence of *H. pylori* and incidence of gastric cancer
- Gastric cancer has declined as the rate of *H. pylori* infection has fallen
- Infected individuals have an increased risk of gastric cancer
- *H. pylori* causes gastric atrophy and intestinal metaplasia that precede dysplasia and neoplasia
- Corporal gastritis increases gastric pH and reduces secretion of vitamin C, predisposing to bacterial proliferation and production of carcinogenic nitroso compounds

impact on gastric cancer is only likely to occur with improved living standards and possibly vaccination.

Gastric lymphoma. In some individuals, *H. pylori* infection induces a proliferation of gastric mucosal lymphocytes. In a very small minority, this progresses to true lymphoma – so-called MALT lymphoma. In most people, the lesion regresses following *H. pylori* eradication. Both gastric cancer and MALT lymphoma are particularly associated with a strain of *H. pylori* that produces a specific toxin called CagA.

Functional dyspepsia. The role of *H. pylori* in dyspepsia in the absence of ulcer disease is probably negligible. Based on the available evidence, summarized below, it is probably of primary importance in only a minority of patients suffering from this heterogeneous disorder.

- Only a minority of those infected have symptoms.
- *H. pylori*-positive patients have dyspepsia symptoms comparable to those of *H. pylori*-negative patients.
- Although dyspeptic patients appear to have a higher prevalence of infection than non-dyspeptics, the control individuals used in many studies have been inappropriate.
- Some patients' symptoms improve after eradication therapy, but other studies have shown no beneficial effect in either ulcer-like or dysmotility-like dyspepsia.

Methods of detection

The advantages, disadvantages and application of tests for *H. pylori* in clinical practice are summarized in Table 3.4.

Rapid urease test. This is usually the *Campylobacter*-like organism (CLO) test, which is performed during endoscopy. Infected biopsies result in ammonia generation and raised pH, changing the indicator from yellow to pink. This is a reliable, routine method of establishing *H. pylori* status.

Histology and culture tend to be reserved for clinical trials. However, culture is also used in areas where antibiotic resistance is common, as antibiotic sensitivities can be determined at the same time.

TABLE 3.4

Tests used in the detection of *H. pylori*

Test	Sensitivity (%)	Specificity (%)	Advantages
Rapid urease test	≤ 95	95	Rapid result
Histology	85	100	Very specific
Culture	95	100	Establishes antibiotic sensitivity
Urea breath test	97	95	Non-invasive
Serology	70–90	50–90	Inexpensive
Fecal test	90	99	Inexpensive

Urea breath test (UBT) is a non-invasive test for establishing current *H. pylori* status (Figure 3.6) and is particularly useful when there is doubt following eradication therapy. The validity of the test is significantly impaired if it is used less than 28 days after completing *H. pylori* eradication or within 14 days of stopping a proton-pump inhibitor.

Serological tests are valuable for population screening, but have little use in post-eradication evaluation because antibody titers may take several months or years to fall. Laboratory-based tests have better specificity and sensitivity than tests promoted for office use.

Fecal antigen tests are now available and have similar applications to the UBT.

Who should be treated?

The meeting of the European *Helicobacter pylori* Study Group in September 2000 strongly recommended eradication in the following circumstances:

- duodenal and gastric ulcer including complicated disease or a confirmed past history
- MALT lymphoma
- following gastric resection for cancer
- those who are first-degree relatives of gastric cancer patients –

Disadvantages	Application
Requires endoscopy	Routine during endoscopy
Requires endoscopy and is expensive	Supplements rapid urease test
Expensive and delay in obtaining results	In areas of high antibiotic resistance
Expensive	To check eradication
Poor specificity (laboratory tests are superior to 'office' kits)	Screening
May encounter patient resistance	To check eradication

because possible predisposing genetic factors may increase the risk of *H. pylori*-induced carcinogenesis

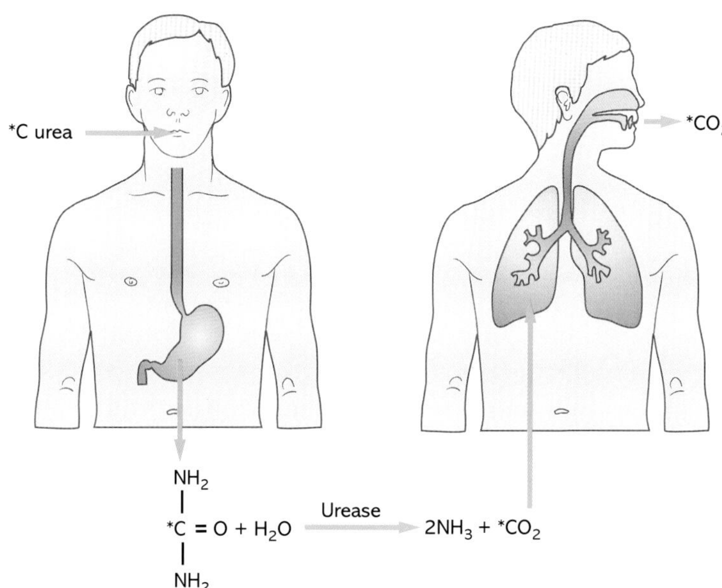

Figure 3.6 The urea breath test. Urea containing a carbon isotope label is given to the patient. If *H. pylori* is present in the stomach, the urea is metabolized and labeled carbon dioxide is detectable in the patient's breath.

- when it is requested by informed and counseled dyspeptic patients.

The meeting also proposed that eradication is an acceptable option in other situations even though irrefutable supporting evidence is currently unavailable. These situations include:

- functional dyspepsia – because long-term relief occurs in a small subgroup of *H. pylori*-positive patients without overt mucosal disease.
- NSAID users. When offering eradication therapy in this group the following facts should be borne in mind.
  - It is impossible to predict in an individual patient whether the drug or the infection is the main etiological factor for dyspepsia or ulceration.
  - *H. pylori* eradication may reduce the risk of ulcers if given before NSAID use.
  - Eradication alone is insufficient to prevent recurrent ulceration in high-risk NSAID users.
  - Eradication does not enhance healing of peptic ulcers in patients on antisecretory therapy continuing to take NSAIDs.
- long-term proton pump inhibition therapy – *H. pylori* has a tendency to migrate from the antrum to the gastric corpus during long-term therapy with these drugs, leading to atrophic gastritis and the subsequent potential risk of gastric ulcer or cancer.

Currently eradication is not recommended for:

- GERD
- asymptomatic subjects.

Patients with gastroesophageal reflux. *H. pylori* infection is not a risk factor for the disease in the great majority of patients with GERD. GERD symptoms and their response to therapy are usually unaffected by *H. pylori* eradication.

Asymptomatic subjects. Treating asymptomatic subjects may potentially prevent progression to peptic ulcer and possibly reverse premalignant gastric mucosal disease. Disadvantages include antibiotic-induced side-effects and the development of resistant strains. Once aware that they are infected, many people, even in the absence of symptoms, will 'demand' eradication therapy, and such requests are often difficult to resist.

Eradication regimens

H. pylori eradication rates of over 90% are now readily achievable. The most extensively studied and consistently effective regimens consist of a proton-pump inhibitor and two antibiotics given for 7 days. Comparable results have also been reported with ranitidine bismuth citrate in combination with clarithromycin and metronidazole or amoxicillin (Table 3.5).

TABLE 3.5

Recommended 7-day, triple-therapy regimens

A

Omeprazole, 20 mg twice a day **or** lansoprazole, 30 mg twice a day **or** pantoprazole, 40 mg twice a day **or** ranitidine bismuth citrate, 400 mg twice a day
PLUS
Metronidazole, 400 mg twice a day
PLUS
Clarithromycin, 250 mg or 500 mg twice a day

B

Omeprazole, 20 mg twice a day **or** lansoprazole, 30 mg twice a day **or** pantoprazole, 40 mg twice a day **or** ranitidine bismuth citrate, 400 mg twice a day
PLUS
Amoxicillin, 1 g twice a day
PLUS
Clarithromycin, 500 mg twice a day

C

Omeprazole, 40 mg once a day **or** lansoprazole, 30 mg twice a day
PLUS
Amoxicillin, 500 mg three times a day
PLUS
Metronidazole, 400 mg three times a day

Helicobacter pylori – Key points

- The prevalence of infection has fallen significantly in the developed world during the past 50 years.
- Infection is closely associated with
  - chronic gastritis
  - peptic ulcer
  - gastric cancer
  - MALT lymphoma.
- Eradication therapy is the most clinically effective and cost-effective means of treating peptic ulcer.

In areas where metronidazole resistance is common, it is logical to use a regimen without this antibiotic or to ascertain bacterial sensitivities before prescribing.

With gastric ulcer, successful eradication can be confirmed at repeat endoscopy. For the majority of other patients, eradication may be assumed if symptoms resolve. For those who continue to be symptomatic and for patients for whom persistent infection would be potentially hazardous (Table 3.6), the UBT is an appropriate means of confirming eradication. When infection persists despite satisfactory compliance, a further course of triple therapy extended for 10 or 14 days should be tried. If proton-pump-inhibitor-based triple therapy fails, an alternative approach would be to use a bismuth-containing regimen (Table 3.7).

So-called 'dual therapy' using a proton-pump inhibitor and a single antibiotic achieves unsatisfactory eradication rates and may encourage bacterial resistance. It is not recommended.

TABLE 3.6

At-risk patients in whom eradication should be confirmed

- History of complicated ulcer
- Long-term anticoagulant medication
- Frail patients with serious concomitant disease

TABLE 3.7

Recommended 14-day regimen after proton-pump inhibitor-based triple-therapy failure

A proton-pump inhibitor, twice a day, with tripotassium dicitrato bismuthate, 120 mg twice a day **or** ranitidine bismuth citrate, 400 mg twice a day
PLUS
Metronidazole, 400 mg three times a day
PLUS
Tetracycline, 500 mg three times a day

Key references

Banatvola N, Mayo K, Megraud F et al. The cohort effect and *Helicobacter pylori. J Infect Dis* 1993;168:219–21.

Blum AL, Talley NJ, O'Morain C et al. Lack of effect of treating *Helicobacter pylori* infection in patients with nonulcer dyspepsia. *N Engl J Med* 1998;339:1875–81.

Dixon MF. *Helicobacter pylori* and peptic ulceration: histopathological aspects. *J Gastroenterol Hepatol* 1991;6:125–30.

Drumm B, Perez-Perez GI, Blaser MJ, Sherman PM. Intrafamilial clustering of *H. pylori* infection. *N Engl J Med* 1990;322:359–63.

Fox JG. Postulated transmission of *H. pylori. Aliment Pharmacol Ther* 1995;9(suppl 2):93–103.

Hulton K, Han SW, Enroth H et al. *Helicobacter pylori* in the drinking water in Peru. *Gastroenterology* 1996;110:1031–5.

Marshall BJ. The 1995 Albert Lasker Medical Research Award. *Helicobacter pylori.* The etiologic agent for peptic ulcer. *JAMA* 1995;274:1064–6.

McColl K, Murray L, El-Omar E *et al.* Symptomatic benefit from eradicating *H. pylori* in patients with nonulcer dyspepsia. *N Engl J Med* 1998;339:1869–74.

Misiewicz JT. Management of *Helicobacter pylori*-related disorders. *Eur J Gastroenterol Hepatol* 1997;9(suppl 1):S17–21.

Nomara A, Stemmermann GV, Chyou PH et al. *Helicobacter pylori* and gastric carcinoma among Japanese Americans in Hawaii. *N Engl J Med* 1991;325:1132–6.

Primary Care Society for Gastroenterology. *Decision points for the management of H. pylori in primary care.* March 1997.

Talley NJ, Janssens J, Lauritsen K et al. Eradication of *H. pylori* in functional dyspepsia – randomised double blind placebo controlled trial with 12 month follow up. *BMJ* 1999;318:833–7.

The Eurogast Study Group. An international association between *H. pylori* infection and gastric cancer. *Lancet* 1993;341:1359–62.

The European *Helicobacter pylori* Study Group. The Maastricht Consensus Report. 2000.

Warren JR, Marshall BJ. Unidentified curved bacilli on gastric epithelium in active chronic gastritis. *Lancet* 1983;i:1273–5.

4 Peptic ulcer

The exact incidence and prevalence of peptic ulcer have always been uncertain because of the remitting and relapsing nature of the disease and the erratic investigation of dyspepsia. A decade ago, the lifetime risk of peptic ulcer in the UK was approximately 10%, and about 500 000 new cases were diagnosed in the USA each year.

Duodenal ulcer is three to four times more common than gastric ulcer. In the past the disease predominated in men, but the male:female ratio now approximates to unity, particularly in the elderly (Figure 4.1).

Although physician visit rates have fallen in the developed world (Figure 4.2) the number of hospitalizations for ulcer hemorrhage has risen. Every year, approximately 2500 people in the UK die from peptic ulcer hemorrhage; of these, more than 90% are over the age of 60 years (Figure 4.3). Without control of the disease, 15% of ulcer patients may experience hemorrhage within 10 years of diagnosis, and it has been estimated that 15% of those who bleed eventually die as a result of their ulcer. Until it was recently established that we could change their natural history by *H. pylori* eradication, duodenal and gastric

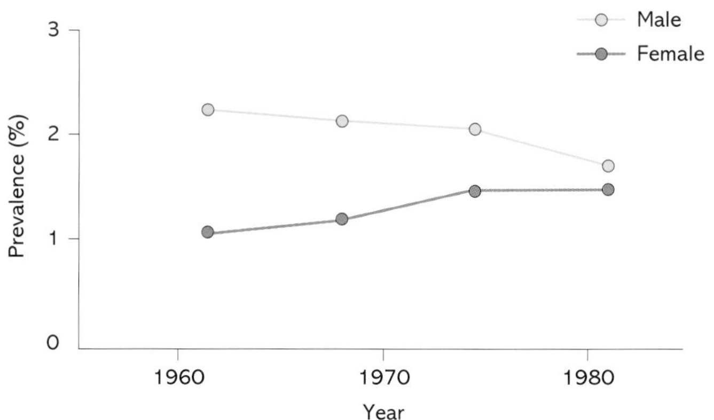

Figure 4.1 The prevalence of peptic ulcer has decreased in males and increased in females. Data from Kurata JH. *Gastroenterology* 1989;96:569–80 and Kurata JH et al. *Am J Public Health* 1985;75:625–9.

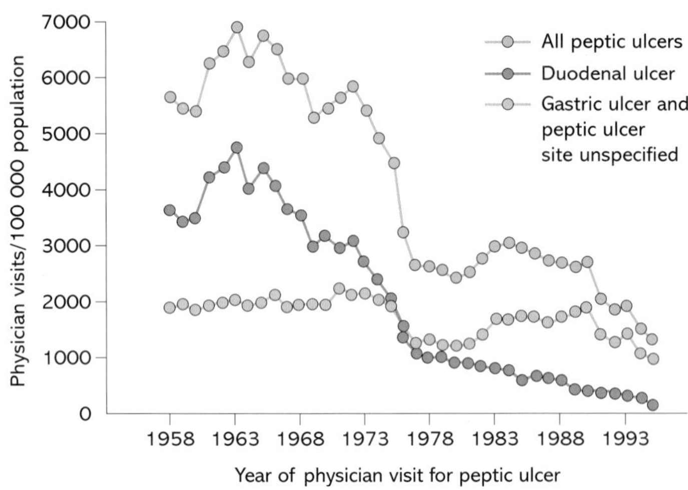

Figure 4.2 Rate of physician visits for peptic ulcer. Derived from Munnangi and Sonnenberg 1997.

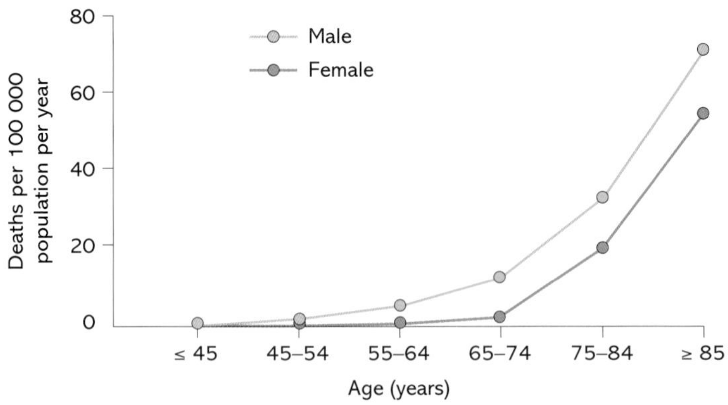

Figure 4.3 Mortality in peptic ulcer disease increases with age. Many older patients with ulcer disease have concomitant cardiorespiratory disease.

ulcers were chronic diseases with annual relapse rates of around 80% and 40%, respectively.

In the Western world, the incidence of peptic ulcer has been in decline for the past 30 years, mainly as a result of the falling prevalence of *H. pylori* infection. It seems likely that this decline will be

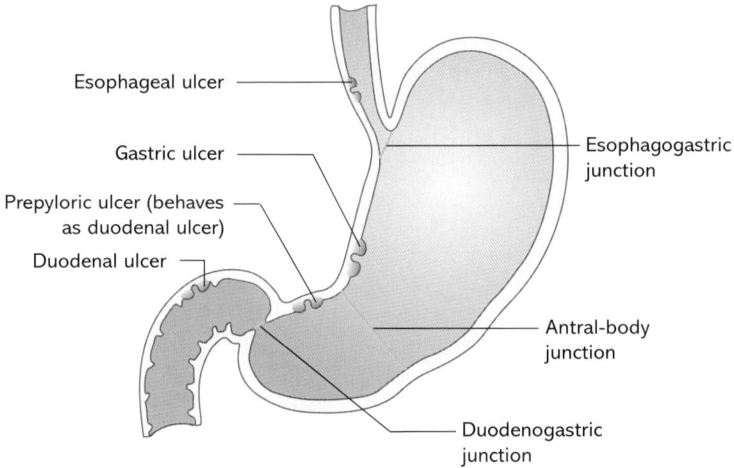

Figure 4.4 Peptic ulcers commonly occur adjacent to mucosal junctions.

accelerated further by the widespread adoption of bacterial eradication, though the increasing use of NSAIDs may be counteractive. By far the most common sites of peptic ulcer are the first part of the duodenum and the stomach (Figure 4.4). Ulcers may also occur in the esophagus as a consequence of gastroesophageal reflux (Chapter 2) and, very rarely, at a gastroenteric stoma following gastric surgery or in association with a Meckel's diverticulum.

Pathogenesis

The traditional view is that peptic ulceration occurs when gastroduodenal mucosa breaks down under the erosive effect of gastric acid and pepsin. The pathogenic factors promoting this imbalance are now known to include:

- *Helicobacter pylori* gastroduodenitis
- defective gastroduodenal mucosal defense (most frequently due to NSAIDs)
- hypergastrinemia and hypersecretion of gastric acid and pepsin
- gastroduodenal dysmotility.

Mucosal defense. The maintenance of mucosal defense (Figure 4.5) depends on many factors, including:

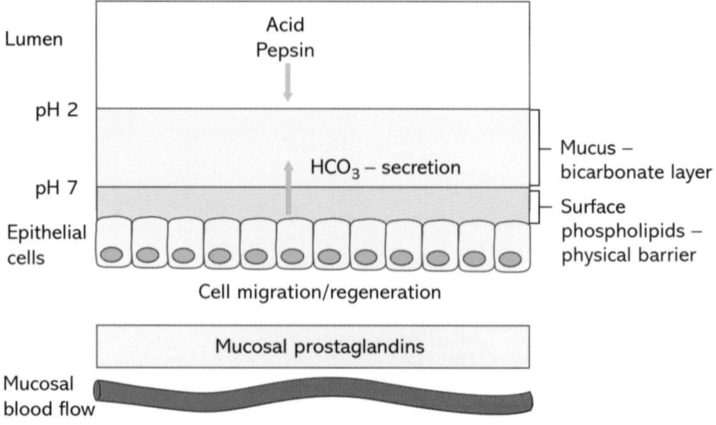

Figure 4.5 Maintenance of mucosal defense. The mucus layer retains bicarbonate, which is secreted by epithelial cells and neutralizes acid as it penetrates from the lumen. The epithelial cells form a second line of defense. Prostaglandin secretion suppresses acid secretion and increases mucosal blood flow, which is essential for epithelial integrity.

- the structure of the epithelial surface and its ability to regenerate and repair
- secretion of water, mucus and bicarbonate
- mucosal blood flow.

At the mucosal level, the pathogenic processes that result in ulceration have still to be clarified. Mucosal integrity is, however, compromised by factors such as *H. pylori* toxins, NSAIDs, corticosteroids and smoking (see Table 4.1).

Helicobacter pylori. Although it is now accepted that *H. pylori* is the predominant etiological factor in duodenal and gastric ulcer (Table 4.1), there are distinct differences in the pathogenesis of the two diseases. Both the direct effect and the location of bacterial inflammation differ, and the impact on acid secretion varies.

Duodenal ulcer. In patients who progress to duodenal ulceration, *H. pylori* infection is confined mainly to the gastric antrum. The mucosa in this portion of the stomach contains gastrin-producing G-cells and somatostatin-secreting D-cells. Gastrin secretion in response

TABLE 4.1

Etiological risk factors and special features of peptic ulcer

H. pylori

- Infection is found in 95% of duodenal ulcer and 80% of gastric ulcer patients

NSAIDs

- Counteract the protective effects of prostaglandins
- Approximately 20% of regular users have ulceration of the gastroduodenal mucosa
- Risk of ulceration is increased by concomitant steroid therapy, smoking and possibly *H. pylori* infection
- Typical pain is often absent
- Presentation with anemia and acute hemorrhage is common
- Toxicity varies according to drug: azapropazone and piroxicam appear to be particularly toxic; ibuprofen and the Cox-2 selective drugs are less so

Smoking

- Smokers have an increased prevalence of ulcers, delayed healing and increased incidence of complications

Steroids

- Long-term use of corticosteroids may increase risk of peptic ulcer, but the risk is lower than that associated with NSAID therapy

Genetic

- Siblings are 2.5 times more likely to have an ulcer compared with controls
- Genetic studies may have been confounded by familial transmission of *H. pylori*

to food stimulates parietal cells in the body of the stomach to produce acid. Somatostatin is secreted in the presence of excess acid; it inhibits gastrin release, thus preventing excessive acid secretion.

H. pylori infection of the antrum leads to the suppression of somatostatin release from D-cells. This causes a rise in gastrin and, in turn, increased secretion of acid by parietal cells, the numbers of which are increased in duodenal ulcer patients (Figure 4.6). This excess acid passes into the duodenum, where it induces gastric metaplasia in the duodenal mucosa. *H. pylori*, which is incapable of infecting healthy duodenal mucosa, now colonizes the patches of gastric metaplasia, leading to duodenitis and ulceration.

Gastric ulcer. In gastric ulcer, antritis is accompanied by inflammation of the gastric body, where it results in atrophy of the mucosa and reduction of acid secretion. These conditions predispose to ulceration in the stomach, but other factors that have yet to be fully identified or confirmed must also be involved.

Non-steroidal anti-inflammatory drugs. The world market for NSAIDs is estimated at US$8 billion, and the cost of treating the adverse GI events due to these drugs is likely to exceed this amount.

Among NSAID users 20% experience GI symptoms, and endoscopic studies have found gastric ulceration in 20% and duodenal ulceration in 8%.

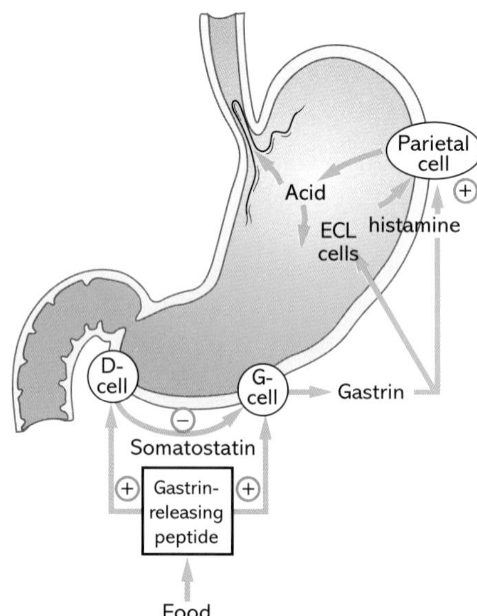

Figure 4.6 The control of acid secretion and the relationship between G-, D- and parietal cells.

The efficacy of NSAIDs depends on the inhibition of the enzyme cyclooxygenase-2 (Cox-2) that converts arachidonic acid to prostaglandins, which are important mediators of inflammatory reactions. However, these same drugs damage the gastroduodenal mucosa by inhibiting the enzyme cyclooxygenase-1 (Cox-1), which is vital for the synthesis of endogenous prostaglandins that regulate the mucosal defenses (Figure 4.5).

Acute injury. Aspirin and the majority of NSAIDs are weak acids that readily penetrate the gastric mucosal barrier and surface epithelium, where release of hydrogen ions directly disrupts the cells. The mucosa is then additionally vulnerable to the other agents such as acid and pepsin, leading to erosion and petechial hemorrhage. With continued usage the mucosa frequently becomes less susceptible to the direct damaging effect of these drugs.

Chronic injury. The chronic ulcerative effects of NSAIDs are not due to the local impact on the mucosa but to the systemic inhibition of prostaglandin synthesis, which impairs mucosal defense by reducing water and bicarbonate secretion, the integrity of the mucus/gel layer and mucosal blood flow.

Recently developed NSAIDs that predominantly inhibit Cox-2 rather than Cox-1 appear to reduce inflammation effectively without damaging the gastroduodenal mucosa.

Gastroduodenal dysmotility. Excessive acidification of the duodenal bulb, and the mucosal damage that results from consequent uncoordinated and rapid gastric emptying, occur in some patients with duodenal ulcer. These factors may constitute the predominant pathogenic mechanism in non-*H. pylori* / non-NSAID duodenal ulcers. The proportion of ulcers in this category has recently increased in the USA.

Duodenogastric reflux of bile and pancreatic enzymes may be supplementary etiological factors in gastric ulcer.

Zollinger–Ellison syndrome. Zollinger–Ellison (ZE) syndrome is a rare cause of duodenal ulcer. It is characterized by a very high basal rate of gastric acid secretion due, in the majority of patients, to a gastrin-producing tumor of the pancreas. The tumor is also found less commonly in other abdominal organs. Rarely, the syndrome results from hyperplasia of G cells in the antrum. The features of ZE syndrome are summarized in Table 4.2.

Diagnosis

Pain localized to the epigastrium is the characteristic feature of peptic ulcer. More rarely, pain occurs in the hypochondria or around the umbilicus. Radiation retrosternally or to the back is often experienced. It is usually described as 'gnawing' or 'knife-like'. Sometimes patients describe a feeling of severe hunger. The pain can last from several minutes to a few hours. Increasing intensity of pain does not indicate incipient perforation or hemorrhage, but may be the result of penetration into the pancreas. Without treatment, pain tends to occur in bouts which persist for a few weeks, followed by remissions which may last for several months. Pain in the early hours is a feature of duodenal ulcer; it is unrelated to eating in at least 50% of patients. Consistent relief with antacids is frequently reported.

Vomiting and reflux. Although uncommon, vomiting that relieves pain is a sensitive indicator of duodenal ulcer. Heartburn and regurgitation also occur frequently.

Examination. The only physical sign of uncomplicated peptic ulcer is epigastric tenderness. The presence of this sign does not discriminate an ulcer from other abdominal diseases.

TABLE 4.2

Features of Zollinger–Ellison syndrome

- Absence of *H. pylori* infection
- Failure of ulcer to heal with routine acid suppression
- Ulceration beyond the first part of the duodenum
- Accompanying diarrhea or steatorrhea
- Response to tumor resection or high-dose proton-pump inhibitor therapy

Importantly, it is not possible to distinguish between gastric and duodenal ulcers on the basis of clinical features alone.

Investigations

Upper gastrointestinal endoscopy is the first choice for patients with symptoms suggestive of peptic ulcer. It is more accurate than a barium meal, allows histological diagnosis and establishes *H. pylori* status. A barium meal should be reserved for patients stating a preference for this procedure or when endoscopy is technically impossible. However, if an initial barium meal shows gastric ulcer, it should be followed by UGI endoscopy to exclude malignancy.

Biochemical tests. Anemia due to occult bleeding should always be excluded in ulcer disease. In ZE syndrome, the serum gastrin level will be greatly elevated and the basal level of acid secretion will be high. Elevated serum gastrin levels are also found in patients taking acid-suppressant drugs and those with pernicious anemia.

Management

***H. pylori*-associated ulcers.** Bacterial eradication therapy is the first choice for newly diagnosed duodenal and gastric ulcers following confirmation of *H. pylori* infection (Chapter 3). It is undoubtedly the most cost-effective means of ulcer management, because successful eradication dramatically reduces recurrence (Figure 4.7).

It is also acceptable to offer eradication therapy to patients with a past history of confirmed chronic ulcer disease, even when *H. pylori* status has not been established. Some physicians, nevertheless, prefer to confirm infection by serology or UBT.

Ulcers heal following successful eradication; prolonged courses of either H_2-receptor antagonists or proton-pump inhibitors are not usually required for uncomplicated disease. However, some patients continue to use them for a few weeks if symptoms persist temporarily.

Confirmation of healing. Repeat endoscopy is unnecessary for patients with uncomplicated duodenal ulcer. Resolution of symptoms can be taken as confirmation of eradication and healing. In contrast,

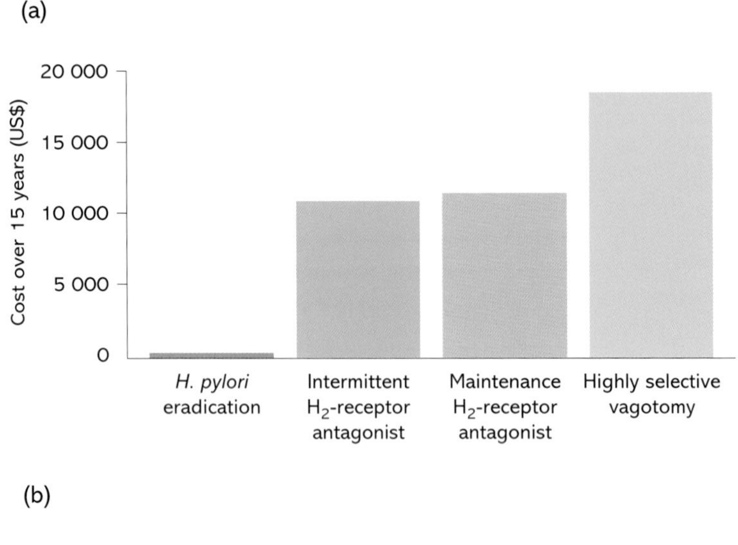

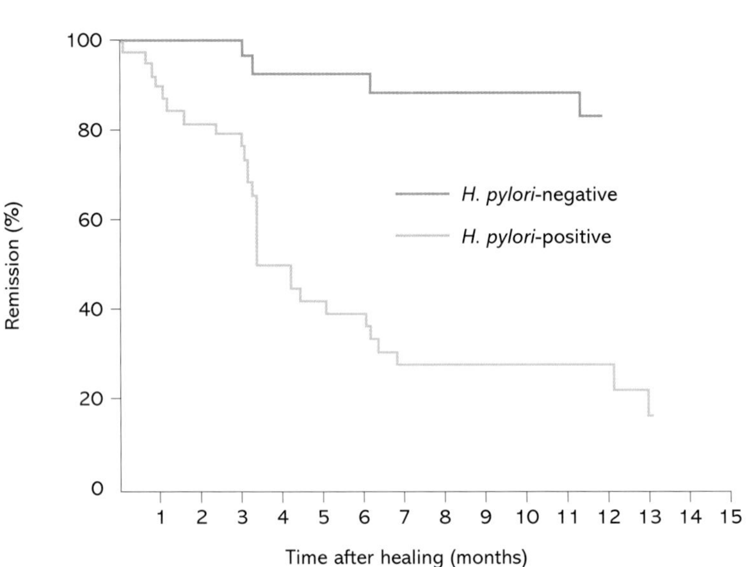

Figure 4.7 (a) Predicted costs of duodenal ulcer management strategies over 15 years (data from Sonnenberg and Townsend 1995); (b) eradication of *H. pylori* dramatically reduces the recurrence of duodenal ulcer. Reproduced with permission from Calam J. *Clinician's Guide to Helicobacter Pylori*. London: Chapman and Hall, 1996.

gastric ulcer healing must be confirmed by repeat endoscopy, which in addition provides the means of reassessing *H. pylori* status.

For duodenal ulcer presenting with hemorrhage or perforation, current practice is to suppress acid secretion for 4 weeks, in addition to giving eradication therapy, to enhance healing. Furthermore, many gastroenterologists recommend endoscopic confirmation of healing and bacterial clearance for this patient group. Successful eradication virtually eliminates the risk of recurrent bleeding.

Persistent symptoms. Dyspepsia that persists after eradication therapy for ulcer disease is rarely due to failed bacterial clearance or continuing ulceration, as eradication rates of over 90% are now readily achievable. Residual symptoms are usually due to coexisting disorders, such as reflux disease or functional dyspepsia (see Chapter 6).

In this circumstance, the UBT is the most sensitive and convenient means of excluding persistent infection. If failed eradication is confirmed, a further antibacterial course should be given (Chapter 3). Failure to eradicate *H. pylori* in ulcer disease leaves the patient at risk of recurrence and potential complications. In this situation, long-term maintenance with acid suppression is the logical means of disease control.

NSAID-associated ulcers. When the NSAID is withdrawn, ulcers heal rapidly on standard acid-suppressant therapy. If the NSAID has to be continued, ulcer healing is slowed when H_2-receptor antagonists are used at routine dosage. Proton-pump inhibition is therefore preferable. Concomitant prophylactic protective therapy should be considered in certain NSAID users (Table 4.3); proton-pump inhibitors are more effective than H_2-receptor antagonists or misoprostol. The promising toxicity profile of Cox-2 selective agents should encourage their use as first-choice drugs in these at-risk patients.

The relationship between *H. pylori* infection and NSAID use is uncertain. The pathogenic mechanisms are distinct and probably act independently.

It is not current practice to establish *H. pylori* status or to offer eradication to NSAID users because there is, at present, no established

TABLE 4.3

Patients using NSAIDs for whom concomitant prophylactic proton-pump inhibitor therapy should be considered

- Patients with previous history of significant dyspepsia symptoms*
- Patients with previous history of ulcer, particularly with complications*
- Smokers*
- Patients receiving a high-dose NSAID or concomitant steroid therapy
- Patients given NSAIDs known to be associated with a higher incidence of gastrointestinal complications, such as piroxicam or azapropazone
- Elderly*

* A logical alternative to prophylactic PPI therapy would be the use of a Cox-2-selective drug.

proof that this would significantly reduce the incidence of NSAID-induced disease or enhance its management.

Non-*H. pylori*, non-NSAID ulcers. Although still in a minority, there is an increasing proportion of chronic peptic ulcers that are not associated with *H. pylori* or NSAID usage. They are suitably controlled by prolonged acid-suppressant therapy.

Endoscopic management of acute hemorrhage. Acute hemorrhage from ulcers accounts for 2500 deaths annually in the UK. In the USA, the reported mortality rate from acute UGI hemorrhage is 5–14% and depends on variables such as age and comorbid conditions.

Early endoscopic examination allows investigation of the bleeding site, which can then be treated by laser, heater probe or injection of adrenaline and sclerosant. Such intervention reduces rates of re-bleeding, transfusion requirements, surgical referral and hospitalization time.

Eradication therapy in *H. pylori*-positive patients significantly reduces the risk of recurrent ulceration and bleeding. By contrast, when bleeding has occurred from a NSAID-associated ulcer and a NSAID is continued long term, proton-pump inhibitor therapy is essential.

Surgery. Increasing use of pharmacological control of gastric acid secretion has accelerated the decline of surgical management of uncomplicated peptic ulcer (Figure 4.8), and it has become virtually obsolete since the introduction of *H. pylori* eradication. The most common indication for surgical intervention is gastric ulcer that fails to heal on medical treatment. This raises the suspicion of undiagnosed malignancy, which is found in approximately 2% of gastric ulcers originally considered to be benign. Most surgeons now opt for minimal intervention when operating for bleeding or perforation because the disease can be managed subsequently by *H. pylori* eradication or long-term acid suppression.

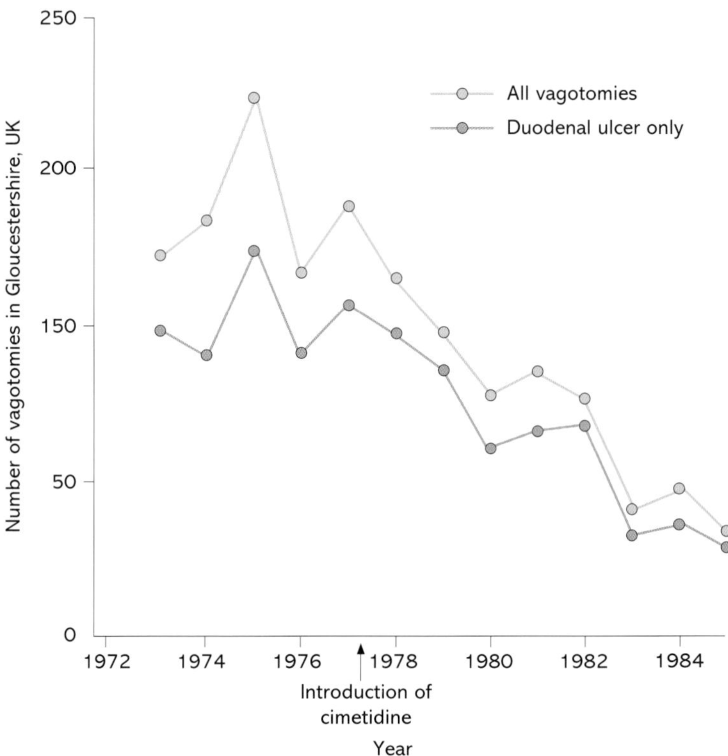

Figure 4.8 The introduction of cimetidine in 1976 resulted in a rapid decline in operations for duodenal ulcer in Gloucestershire, UK. Reproduced from Gear MWL 1986.

Peptic ulcer – Key points

- The incidence of duodenal and gastric ulcer due to *H. pylori* continues to fall in the developed world.
- Non-*H.-pylori*-associated peptic ulcer is now the commonest cause of complicated ulcer disease in the developed world.
- Persistent or recurrent symptoms after appropriate eradication therapy are unusually due to continuing infection or ulceration.

Key references

Baron JH. Peptic ulcer: a problem almost solved. *J R Coll Physicians Lond* 1997;31:512–20.

Bjorkman DJ. Current status of nonsteroidal anti-inflammatory drug (NSAID) use in the United States: risk factors and frequency of complications. *Am J Med* 1999;107(6a):35–105.

Gabriel SE, Jaakkimainen L, Bombardier C. Risk of serious gastrointestinal complications related to the use of non-steroidal anti-inflammatory drugs: a meta-analysis. *Ann Int Med* 1991;115:787–96.

Gear MWL. The place of surgery in the management of peptic ulcer. A comparison with modern drug therapy. In: Lancaster Smith MJ, ed. *Peptic Ulcer*. London: Update Siebert, 1986.

Graham DY, Hepps KS, Ramirez FC et al. Treatment of *Helicobacter pylori* reduces the rate of re-bleeding in peptic ulcer disease. *Scand J Gastroenterol* 1993;28:939–42.

Hall AS, Lauritsen AH, Dalsguard V et al. Non steroidal anti-inflammatory drugs and upper gastrointestinal bleeding. Identifying high risk groups by excess risk estimates. *Scand J Gastroenterol* 1995;30:438–44.

Hawkey LJ. COX-2 inhibition. *Lancet* 1999;353:307–14.

Jaspersen D. Helicobacter eradication: the best long-term prophylaxis for ulcer bleeding recurrence? *Endoscopy* 1995;27: 622–5.

Laine L, Hopkins RJ, Girardi LS. Has the impact of *H. pylori* therapy on ulcer recurrence in the United States been overstated? A meta-analysis of rigorously designed trials. *Am J Gastroenterol* 1998;93: 1409–15.

Munnangi S, Sonnenberg A. Time trends of physician visits and treatment patterns of peptic ulcer disease in the United States. *Arch Int Med* 1997;157:1489–94.

McColl KEL. Pathophysiology of duodenal ulcer disease. *Eur J Gastroenterol* 1997;9(suppl 1): S9–12.

Although UGI symptoms suggestive of esophageal or gastric cancer naturally raise concern in general practice, malignancy is in fact a relatively rare cause of dyspepsia in most of the developed world. Only approximately 3% of all patients investigated by UGI endoscopy in the UK have carcinoma of the esophagus or stomach.

UGI malignancy is particularly rare in young people. A survey by Lancaster Smith in 2001 of 9223 unselected patients consecutively referred from general practitioners to an open-access endoscopy service revealed that:

- the incidences of both esophageal and gastric carcinomas were 1 per 2700 in patients under 45 years of age
- only 1.2% of all patients with carcinoma of the esophagus and 1.5% of those with stomach cancer were below the age of 45.

All of the young patients with malignant disease had one or more of the alarm symptoms (page 66) at the time of referral.

Carcinoma of the esophagus

The incidence of esophageal cancer varies widely; for example, in some areas of China and Iran it exceeds that of Western Europe and North America by a factor of 10. In the USA, incidence is three to four times greater in blacks than in whites. The annual incidence in the UK is approximately 8 per 100 000. The increasing incidence of distal carcinoma in the developed world during the past 30 years is thought to be related to severe gastroesophageal reflux.

Etiopathogenesis. The etiological factors involved include:

- smoking
- heavy consumption of alcohol
- diet (fungal contamination of food; vitamin, iron and zinc deficiencies; high nitrite and nitrate intake)
- Barrett's esophagus / severe gastroesophageal reflux
- achalasia

- celiac disease
- tylosis (familial hyperkeratosis).

Proximal carcinomas are predominantly squamous cell lesions, and those occurring distally are most commonly adenocarcinomas. The incidence of the latter, having increased over the past 20 years, has now reached parity with the former. Esophageal cancer invades the mediastinum and may also extend into the proximal stomach. Lymphatic spread may involve the supraclavicular and intra-abdominal nodes.

Diagnosis and management. The predominant symptom is progressive dysphagia, usually accompanied by some degree of anorexia and weight loss. Upper gastrointestinal endoscopy is the most accurate means of confirming the diagnosis. Staging of the disease by CT, MRI, or increasingly with the aid of endoscopic ultrasound, enables the surgeon to select patients for palliative or potentially curative surgery. The overall 5-year survival in such cases is 10–20%.

Radiotherapy is preferred for upper-third lesions and may be curative. Elsewhere radiotherapy is usually palliative. The primary objective of palliation is to maintain swallowing. New chemotherapeutic regimens have also shown encouraging results in terms of palliation. Other palliative measures include:

- regular endoscopic dilatation
- endoscopically or radiologically positioned stents
- tumor ablation with alcohol or laser.

Improved outcome in the future will depend upon earlier investigation and screening of high-risk patients, such as those with dysplastic Barrett's mucosa and possibly those with severe prolonged gastroesophageal reflux.

Carcinoma of the stomach

Prevalence rates for carcinoma of the stomach vary widely throughout the world. It is particularly common in Japan, Chile, Finland and parts of China. In the developed world, the incidence of cancers in the distal stomach has fallen dramatically during the past 50 years. In contrast, there has been a steady increase in the frequency of proximal carcinomas (Figure 5.1). In the UK, a family physician with an average list will see one new case every 2 years.

Etiopathogenesis. The etiology of the disease involves both genetic and environmental factors (Table 5.1), but there is now little doubt that *H. pylori* is the most important factor in distal lesions (see Chapter 3). The reduced incidence of distal stomach cancer in developed countries has been attributed to the ever-decreasing prevalence of *H. pylori* gastritis. Carcinomas occur in any area of the stomach and may be ulcerative, polypoid or occasionally diffusely infiltrative (linitis plastica). The regional lymph nodes and peritoneum are sites of local spread, with secondary deposits common in the liver and more distant metastases occurring in bone and lung.

Diagnosis and management. The clinical features of gastric cancer include these 'alarm symptoms':

- epigastric pain
- anorexia
- weight loss
- vomiting
- dysphagia
- anemia.

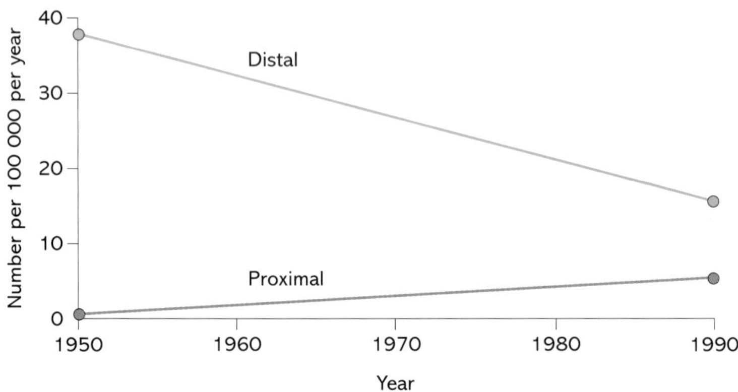

Figure 5.1 Incidence of distal and proximal gastric cancer in The Netherlands. Reproduced with permission from Kuipers EJ 1999.

TABLE 5.1

Etiological factors for carcinoma of the stomach

- *H. pylori* gastritis
- Autoimmune atrophic gastritis – pernicious anemia
- Dietary factors (pickled food, low vitamin / high salt intake, smoked food)
- High nitrate ingestion (contaminated water)
- Previous partial gastrectomy
- Blood group A

Ascites, hepatomegaly and supraclavicular lymphadenopathy are signs of advanced disease. Diagnosis is confirmed by endoscopy and pre-operative staging by CT and laparoscopy.

In Japan, where the incidence of stomach cancer is high, screening programs detect disease at an early stage and 5-year survival rates have risen to 40%. Unfortunately, in the UK, despite the widespread availability of open-access endoscopy, only 50% of patients have resectable tumors and 5-year survival rates range from 7% to 16%.

Adjuvant chemotherapeutic regimens are under investigation and appear to extend survival.

Carcinoma of the esophagus and stomach – Key points

- In developed countries esophageal and gastric cancers are extremely rare in patients under 45.
- The incidence of esophageal and proximal gastric cancer is increasing in those over 45.
- The incidence of distal gastric cancer is decreasing with the fall in the prevalence of *H. pylori* infection.

Key references

Blot WJ, Derassa SS, Kneller RW et al. Rising incidence of carcinoma of the esophagus and gastric cardia. *JAMA* 1991;265:1287–9.

Kuipers EJ. Review: Exploring the link between *H. pylori* and gastric cancer. *Aliment Pharmacol Ther* 1999;13(suppl 1):3–11.

Lagergren J, Bergstrom R, Lindgren A et al. Symptomatic gastroesophageal reflux as a risk factor for esophageal carcinoma. *N Engl J Med* 1999;340:825–31.

6 Functional dyspepsia

Functional dyspepsia refers to discomfort or pain centered in the epigastrium; it may be 'ulcer-like' or 'dysmotility-like'. Ulcer-like dyspepsia is a burning epigastric discomfort or pain that often occurs at night and improves after eating. Dysmotility-like dyspepsia encompasses a sensation of fullness, nausea or bloating, and vomiting. Symptoms are typically worse in the postprandial period.

The word 'functional' indicates that common or uncommon structural disorders, biochemical abnormalities and infectious agents have been excluded by various tests from the etiology of the dyspepsia. As described in Chapter 1, uninvestigated symptoms may be due to many causes. In the absence of alarm symptoms, empirical treatment often resolves the symptoms and they do not return.

However, if alarm symptoms are present or if empirical treatment of a reasonable duration does not relieve the symptoms, the patient should undergo investigation. A more specific diagnosis benefits both patient and physician, leading to:

- a better understanding of the patient's symptoms
- an appreciation of the prognosis for the symptoms
- more specific and rational therapies.

This chapter reviews an approach to the diagnosis and treatment of functional dyspepsia that begins when the common diagnoses responsible for dyspepsia symptoms have been excluded and the symptoms remain unexplained.

Epidemiology

Dyspepsia symptoms are very common and affect 7–40% of various populations. Many patients with mild symptoms do not seek medical attention. The precise number of patients seeking medical care is unknown because of variation in classification. It is clear, however, that in many patients who undergo investigation for dyspepsia symptoms no specific abnormalities are found. For example, approximately 30% of patients undergoing UGI endoscopy for dyspepsia symptoms have normal endoscopic evaluations. Therefore, from a gastroenterologist's viewpoint, approximately 30% of patients with dyspepsia symptoms have functional dyspepsia, provided other causes, such as biliary and pancreatic disease and irritable bowel syndrome, have been excluded.

The definition of functional dyspepsia has been troublesome for many years – dyspepsia literally means 'bad digestion'. The problem stems from the fact that the term is poorly understood by physicians and patients alike – patients do not complain of 'dyspepsia'. Furthermore, the patient may have a difficult time describing the uncomfortable abdominal sensations that they experience after a meal. When physicians try to communicate about dyspepsia, the term is often confused with GERD, heartburn, peptic ulcers, and conditions of mucosal inflammation or ulceration of the esophagus, stomach and/or duodenum.

When standard tests, such as radiographic studies of the UGI tract and upper endoscopy, exclude the common causes of dyspepsia symptoms, disorders of gastric neuromusculature (motility) should be diagnosed and treated appropriately (see below). These abnormalities of motility or the neuromuscular functions of the stomach and duodenum include disorders of:

- fundic and antral contractility and relaxation
- gastric myoelectrical activity
- gastric emptying
- visceral hypersensitivities related to the stomach.

Pathophysiology

Normal postprandial gastroduodenal motility. Myenteric neurons of the enteric nervous system are organized in plexuses between the muscle layers. The fundus relaxes after each swallow via non-adrenergic, non-cholinergic neural pathways that involve nitric oxide. The fundus and proximal body of the stomach relax to receive ingested food, a process called receptive relaxation (Figure 6.1), allowing the stomach to accommodate the volume of ingested food without producing excessive intragastric pressure.

In humans, the gastric peristaltic waves that move food to the gastric body and antrum occur at a rate of 3 per minute. Food is mixed with

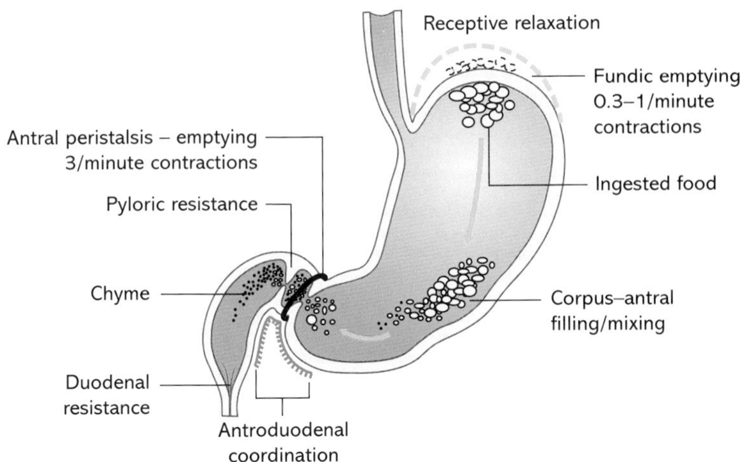

Figure 6.1 Gastric neuromuscular activity in response to a solid meal.

acid and pepsin until the particles (now under 1 mm in size) are in a nutrient suspension called chyme. Waves of antral peristaltic contraction empty 3–4 mL of chyme at a time into the duodenum. Gastric emptying requires coordination of motility between the antrum, pylorus and duodenum.

Normal gastric emptying of solids includes a lag phase lasting 30–45 minutes, depending on the calorie content of the meal, and a linear phase of emptying during which the stomach steadily empties the meal over 2–4 hours, depending on the energy density of the food.

Coordination of gastric peristaltic contractions is by gastric slow waves or pacesetter potentials (Figure 6.2). Pacesetter potentials originate on the greater curvature of the stomach near the junction of the fundus and the proximal corpus. They are electrical depolarization and repolarization wave fronts that migrate circumferentially and distally towards the pylorus at a frequency of 3 cycles per minute (range 2.5–3.7 cpm). The 3-cpm pacesetter potential controls the normal gastric peristaltic waves.

Gastric pacesetter potentials do not produce strong gastric contractions. Circular muscle contraction occurs during action potentials. When the action potentials are linked to the pacesetter potential, coordinated gastric peristaltic waves are propagated from the corpus through the antrum to the pylorus (Figure 6.2). Thus, normal gastric contractility and normal gastric emptying rates are produced by the myoelectrical events of the stomach pacesetter and action potentials.

The origin of the pacesetter potentials remains an area of active investigation. The site of the intrinsic rhythmicity of the stomach appears to be located in the interstitial cells of Cajal. These are specialized cells with properties of neural and smooth muscle elements. The cells are laid out in a meshwork between the longitudinal and circular muscle layers of the stomach and are in close proximity to the myenteric neurons and circular smooth muscle cells.

Abnormalities of the electrical and contractile elements described above may develop in regions of the stomach ranging from the fundus to the body to the antrum and duodenum (Figure 6.3). For example, fundic relaxation in response to ingestion of food may be either excessive or insufficient and result in abnormal fundic relaxation, which is associated with bloating. Antral hypomotility may result from

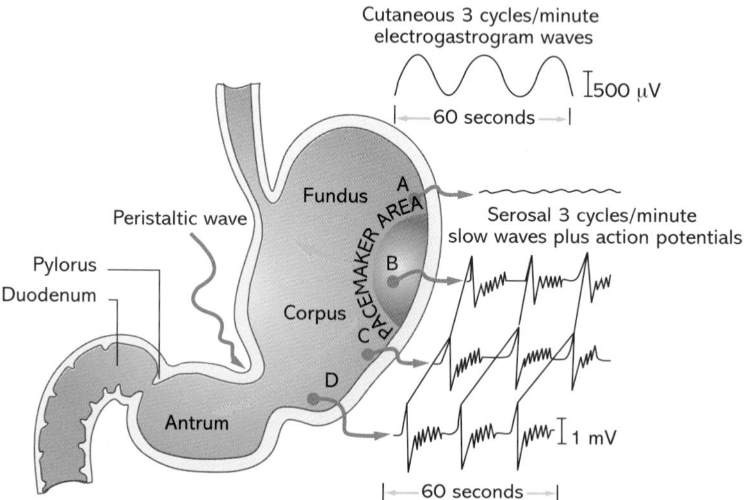

Figure 6.2 Slow waves or pacesetter potentials arise from the pacemaker area. Action potentials and pacesetter potentials are linked to corpus and antral circular muscle contraction, and form the electrical basis of the antral peristaltic wave. A, B, C and D are serosal electrodes.

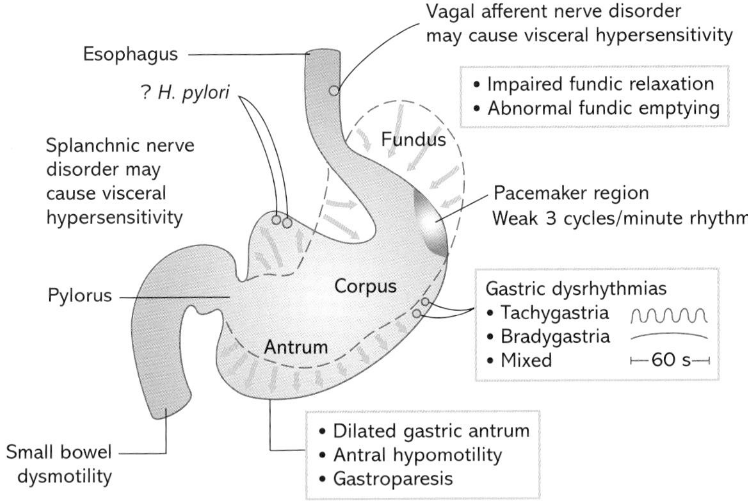

Figure 6.3 Spectrum of neuromuscular dysfunction in dyspepsia. Reproduced with permission from Koch KL, Stern R. *Semin Gastrointest Dis* 1996;4:185–95.

abnormal gastric pacesetter activity or abnormal action-potential activity, both of which may disrupt normal postprandial contractions and emptying rates.

Gastroparesis, or delayed gastric emptying, is the most extreme form of gastric neuromuscular dysfunction. In this situation, a standard meal is not emptied within the range of normal emptying times. In patients with functional dyspepsia defined by vague epigastric discomfort, the incidence of gastroparesis ranges from 20% to 50%. In many patients, viral gastroenteritis or flu-like illness precedes the gastroparesis. Causes of the condition are summarized in Table 6.1.

Gastric dysrhythmias are often found in patients with delayed gastric emptying. They are described as tachygastrias, in which abnormal electrical frequencies range from 3.75 to 10.0 cpm, or bradygastrias (high amplitude or low amplitude), in which abnormal frequencies range from 1.0 to 2.5 cpm (Figure 6.3). Mixed dysrhythmias have elements of both tachygastria and bradygastria.

Gastric dysrhythmias have been recorded in adults and children with dyspepsia symptoms and normal gastric emptying. A recent study

TABLE 6.1

Causes of gastroparesis*

Mechanical obstruction
- Pylorus
- Duodenum
- Small intestine

Postgastric surgery
- Vagotomy
- Antrectomy
- Roux-en-Y
- Fundoplication

Metabolic/endocrine disorders
- Diabetes mellitus
- Hypothyroidism
- Hyperthyroidism
- Adrenal insufficiency

Medications
- Anticholinergic agents
- Narcotics
- L-dopa
- Progesterone
- Estrogen
- Calcium-channel blockers

Mesenteric ischemia

Psychogenic disorders
- Anorexia nervosa
- Bulimia

Smooth-muscle disorders
- Hollow-viscus myopathy
- Scleroderma
- Muscular dystrophy

Neuropathic disorders
- Hollow-viscus neuropathy
- Parkinson's disease
- Paraneoplastic syndrome
- Shy–Drager syndrome

Postviral gastroparesis

Idiopathic disorders
- Idiopathic gastroparesis with gastric dysrhythmia

*Modified from Koch 1997

showed that 60% of patients with dysmotility-like dyspepsia have gastric dysrhythmias. Gastric dysrhythmias are one of the pathophysiological mechanisms associated with postprandial symptoms in these patients. Some patients have a poor 3 cpm postprandial response. The association is supported by the finding that resolution of gastric dysrhythmias and establishment of a normal 3-cpm gastric electrical rhythm is associated with symptom improvement during treatment with domperidone or cisapride.

Disordered intragastric distribution of meals. Patients with dyspepsia have decreased fundal compliance, and ingested meals are moved into the antrum sooner after the meal compared with controls. The altered intragastric movement of food may also evoke dyspepsia symptoms. Distension of the antrum with balloons evokes nausea and gastric dysrhythmias in healthy subjects.

Antral dilatation. Ultrasound studies have shown that the antrum is dilated in patients with functional dysmotility-type dyspepsia. The extent of dilatation correlates with the intensity of bloating symptoms.

Gastric hypersensitivity. Patients with dyspepsia experience discomfort and pain at significantly lower volumes of intragastric balloon distension compared with healthy control subjects. Compliance measures of the fundus, however, are similar in both groups. These findings suggest that the dyspeptic patient may have a 'visceral hypersensitivity' to distension of the stomach. In addition, the fundus does not relax normally in response to duodenal distension in functional dyspepsia, a finding that suggests duodenogastric reflexes are abnormal.

H. pylori. The perceived role of *H. pylori* as a causative agent in dysmotility-like dyspepsia continues to decrease. Recent meta-analysis studies show that eradication therapy in patients with dyspepsia symptoms and *H. pylori* infection results in no significant symptom improvement compared with placebo treatment.

Hormones. Dyspepsia symptoms are often worse premenstrually. Neuromuscular function of the stomach may be affected by the levels of hormones related to the menstrual cycle. Estrogen and progesterone evoke nausea and gastric dysrhythmias in healthy women. The release of hormones may further worsen subtle neuromuscular abnormalities of the stomach and create additional symptoms at these times.

Stress. Acute and chronic physical or psychological stresses or history of abuse may also affect the autonomic nervous system, alter neural hormonal secretions and ultimately affect gastric neuromuscular activities. Studies have shown that patients with chronic dyspepsia do not have obvious psychological profiles or psychiatric disorders. However, anxiety and somatization are present in patients with dysmotility-type chronic dyspepsia.

Clinical presentation

Clinicians should focus on the predominant symptom the patient identifies. If this is epigastric pain, then ulcer-like dyspepsia is the most appropriate diagnosis. If the range of symptoms includes mainly postprandial bloating, fullness, early satiety, nausea and vomiting, a diagnosis of dysmotility-like dyspepsia is better. Symptoms of dysmotility-like dyspepsia may be present during the fasted state, but they usually increase postprandially. Patients often feel poorly after they eat and so modify their diet to minimize symptoms. For the diagnosis of functional dyspepsia, standard diagnostic tests should be normal and symptoms must have been present for 3 months or more (Rome II definitions, Table 6.2).

Diagnosis of functional dyspepsia

The diagnosis of ulcer-like or dysmotility-like functional dyspepsia requires that standard diseases and disorders are excluded. As mentioned previously, the symptoms of dyspepsia are non-specific and therefore GERD, peptic ulcer disease, irritable bowel syndrome, and biliary and pancreatic diseases must be excluded.

Acid peptic diseases, such as GERD, gastric or duodenal ulcer disease, often have some element of a 'burning' sensation in the epigastrium. If the sensation rises into the substernal area, GERD may be diagnosed. Some patients with GERD also have gastric motility disorders, an overlap syndrome that defines dysmotility-like dyspepsia *and* GERD symptoms.

Organic disease often occurs in patients with chronic dyspepsia. In a recent study:

- 24% of patients had GERD
- 21% had gastritis or duodenitis

TABLE 6.2

Rome II definition of functional dyspepsia

Symptoms

Ulcer-like dyspepsia

- Pain centered in the upper abdomen is the predominant (most bothersome) symptom

Dysmotility-like dyspepsia

- An unpleasant or troublesome non-painful sensation (discomfort) centered in the upper abdomen is the predominant symptom; this sensation may be characterized by or associated with upper abdominal fullness, early satiety, bloating, or nausea

Unspecified (non-specific) dyspepsia

- Symptomatic patients whose symptoms do not fulfil the criteria for ulcer-like or dysmotility-like dyspepsia.

Diagnosis

At least 12 weeks, which need not be consecutive, within the preceding 12 months of:

- Persistent or recurrent dyspepsia (pain or discomfort centered in the upper abdomen); and
- No evidence of organic disease (including at upper endoscopy) that is likely to explain the symptoms; and
- No evidence that dyspepsia is exclusively relieved by defecation or associated with the onset of a change in the stool frequency or stool form (i.e., not irritable bowel).

from Talley et al. 1999.

- 20% had peptic ulcer disease
- 2% had gastrointestinal cancer.

Thus, 67% of patients had specific and accepted diagnoses after investigation, even though they had presented with non-specific dyspeptic symptoms. In this series, 33% of the symptomatic patients remained without a specific diagnosis.

Biliary and pancreatic disease. Chronic cholecystitis may also present with non-specific symptoms of postprandial discomfort, bloating and nausea. Pain or discomfort due to biliary diseases is often exacerbated by meals. In a questionnaire study it was found that, of the patients with 'dyspepsia':

- 30% had irritable bowel syndrome
- 29% had GERD
- 25% had a combination of irritable bowel syndrome and gastroesophageal reflux.

Only 6% had gallstones. It is unclear whether or not the gallstones were related to the predominant symptoms reported by the patient.

It may be difficult to determine the relevance of gallstones to a pain syndrome described by an individual patient. If the gallbladder wall is thickened or edematous on ultrasound examination, the evidence suggests chronic inflammation. A gallbladder-emptying study may also indicate disordered contractile function of the gallbladder, a finding associated with chronic cholecystitis.

Chronic pancreatitis is usually accompanied by a moderate-to-severe pain in the epigastrium that radiates into the back. In the presence of increased lipase or amylase, this is not a difficult diagnosis to confirm. More difficult are diagnoses of biliary stenosis or sphincter of Oddi spasm, which may also present with right upper quadrant or with gastric postprandial discomfort.

Small bowel disorders and chronic mesenteric ischemia. In the postprandial period, mesenteric blood flow increases and the small intestine enters a postprandial contractile phase. The small bowel may contribute to postprandial symptoms if strictures, adhesions or narrowings create a bowel obstruction. Small bowel lesions can be subtle and difficult to detect.

Chronic mesenteric ischemia may be due to atherosclerotic disease, intimal hyperplasia or aneurysmal damage to two of the three major abdominal vessels. The ischemic discomfort is usually increased in the postprandial period, but it may be a mild, nondescript pain. Chronic mesenteric ischemia should be considered in the differential diagnosis of dysmotility-like dyspepsia. Symptoms and gastroparesis resolve with vascular bypass surgery.

Standard tests

The approach for an uninvestigated dyspepsia patient is described in Chapter 1. If dyspepsia symptoms have not responded to initial empirical therapy or if there are alarm symptoms, the following clinical approach is suggested to investigate the symptoms.

First, have empirical treatments of GERD, peptic ulcer disease or a neuromuscular abnormality of the stomach been carried out? This usually involves 3–6 weeks of an appropriate drug, such as an H_2-receptor antagonist, proton-pump inhibitor or a promotility agent. Such an approach assumes that there are no alarm features.

Second, if the patient does not respond or if alarm symptoms are present, a UGI series or a UGI endoscopy is the appropriate first step in evaluation (see Figure 6.4, Step 1). The UGI series will exclude:

- gross reflux of gastric content into the esophagus
- large ulcers
- gross obstruction at the antrum, pylorus or duodenum.

Upper gastrointestinal endoscopy will detect these findings and more subtle signs of esophagitis, gastritis or duodenitis. Antral biopsies can also be obtained to determine whether or not *H. pylori* infection is present.

Third, if studies of the esophagus, stomach and duodenum are normal, an ultrasound examination of the gallbladder should be performed. This will exclude cholelithiasis and evidence of gallbladder or peri-gallbladder inflammation. Dilatation of the common bile duct or cystic duct can also be established. Although bowel gas frequently obscures the view, ultrasound may also identify the pancreas and rule out significant pancreatic inflammation, pseudocysts or other retroperitoneal abnormalities that might be associated with the dyspepsia symptoms.

Fourth, if imaging studies plus routine blood studies fail to identify a common or uncommon structural, biochemical or infectious cause of the symptoms, a diagnosis of functional dyspepsia can be made.

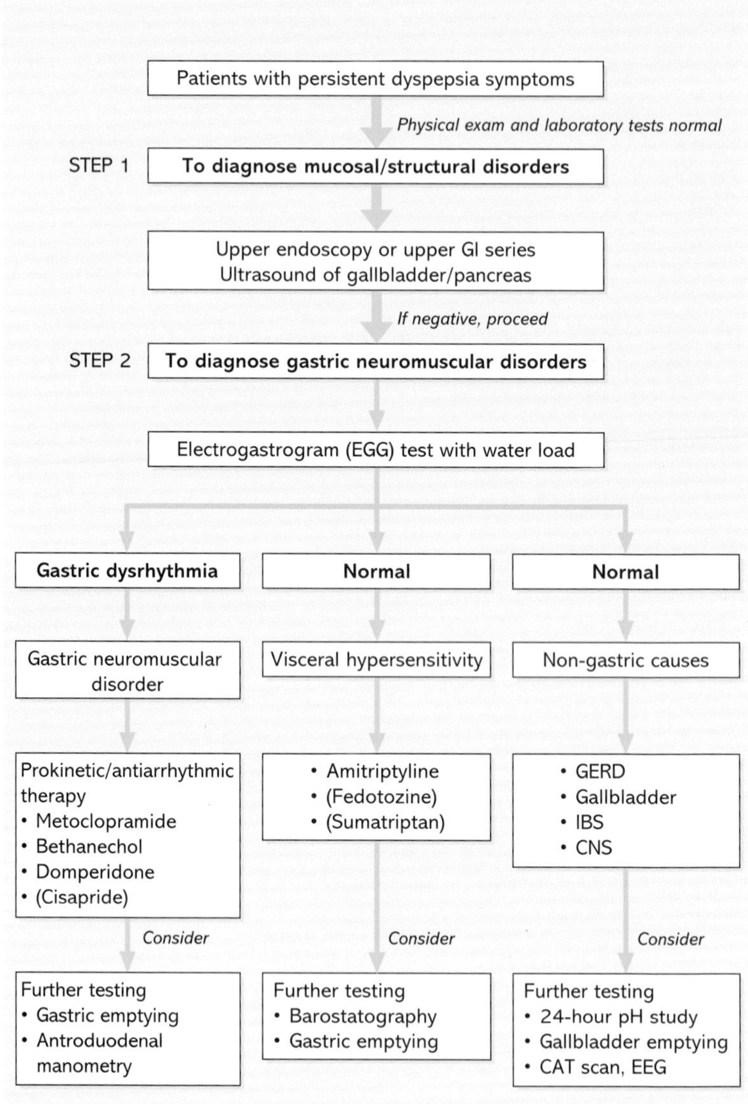

Figure 6.4 An approach to persistent dyspepsia symptoms. Step 1 includes standard tests to diagnose mucosal or structural disorders. If these tests are normal, then Step 2 includes tests to diagnose gastric neuromuscular disorders (or non-gastric disorders) in those patients with persistent and unexplained dyspepsia symptoms.

Unfortunately, investigation of the patient with dysmotility-like dyspepsia frequently ends after a normal endoscopy and/or normal ultrasound are obtained. A diagnostic work-up should continue beyond endoscopy and should address gastric neuromuscular function. A number of non-invasive and invasive tests of gastric motility are available; each test measures a different aspect of gastric neuromuscular activity (Table 6.3).

Non-invasive tests for gastric neuromuscular (motility) abnormalities. Diagnostic methods to measure aspects of gastric motility vary in the level of radiation to which the patient is exposed, invasiveness and time required to perform the test.

Electrogastrography is a non-invasive technique for recording gastric electrical activity. Electrodes are placed on the abdominal surface in the epigastrium, and the electrogastrogram (EGG) reflects the myoelectrical rhythms of the stomach, much as an ECG reflects electrical rhythms of the heart. The normal gastric myoelectrical rhythm is 3 cpm (range 2.5–3.75 cpm) and the rhythm detected by the EGG is similar to the pacesetter potential frequencies recorded by serosal or mucosal electrodes. Abnormal rhythms include bradygastrias (flatline or 1.0–2.5 cpm), tachygastrias and tachyarrhythmias (3.75–10.0 cpm) (Figure 6.5). Duodenal and respiratory frequency rates range from 10 to 15 cpm. Gastric dysrhythmias have been detected in a variety of clinical and research situations in which nausea is a prominent

TABLE 6.3

Gastric motility tests

Test	Result
Solid/liquid gastric emptying (nuclear medicine)	Global stomach function
Electrogastrography	Gastric dysrhythmia
Gastric ultrasound	Antral dilatation
Gastric barostatography	Relaxation/contraction of fundus
Gastroduodenal manometry	Intraluminal pressures in antrum, duodenum, small bowel

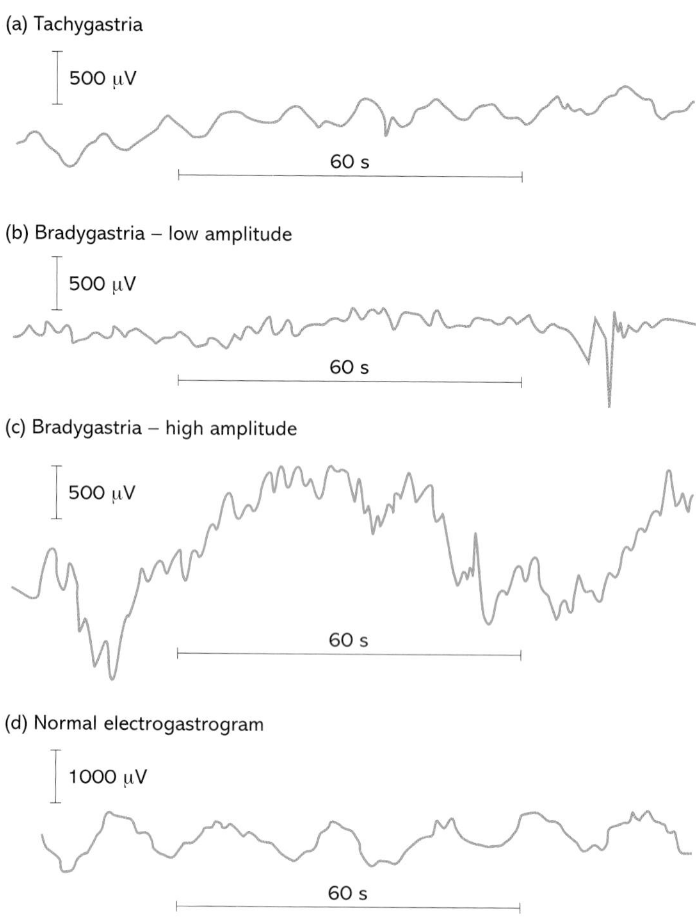

Figure 6.5 Examples of tachygastria, bradygastrias and normal 3 cycle/minute gastric myoelectrical patterns recorded by electrogastrography methods.

symptom, including dysmotility-like dyspepsia, types 1 and 2 diabetes mellitus and nausea of pregnancy.

Gastric emptying tests are usually performed in nuclear medicine departments. The test food is labeled with an isotope and the isotope is identified within the stomach with a gamma camera. The number of counts from the region of interest is calculated over time and expressed as a percentage of the meal emptied or retained. A gastric-emptying curve is constructed that reflects the rate of gastric emptying of the test meal. The test exposes the patient to the approximate equivalent of one or two abdominal radiograph films. Although gastroparesis is diagnosed by this test, the underlying mechanism is not determined. Intragastric distribution of food can also be assessed.

Gastric ultrasound. The antral diameter is measured at several time points after ingestion of standard liquid meals. The rate of gastric emptying is estimated from changes in the antral diameter.

Invasive tests for gastric neuromuscular disorders.

Gastric barostatography. A gastric barostat is a balloon device, mounted on catheters, which is passed into the stomach via the mouth. The balloon is inflated slightly to reflect basal pressure. Subsequent changes in fundic pressure or tone are indicated by changes in the balloon volume as air is either expelled from the balloon or infused into the balloon to maintain the constant basal pressure.

Gastroduodenal manometry. Perfused catheters or solid-phase pressure transducers mounted on flexible catheters are positioned fluoroscopically in the gastric antrum and duodenum to measure intraluminal pressures. Intraluminal pressure changes are registered only if the stomach or duodenal muscle wall contracts to obliterate the lumen; contractions that do not occlude the lumen are not measured. Gastroduodenal manometry tests are invasive and require 10–30 seconds of fluoroscopy time to determine the tube's position.

Gastric neuromuscular evaluation for unexplained functional dyspepsia symptoms

Gastric neuromuscular disorders may be diagnosed by means of non-invasive tests of gastric myoelectrical activity and gastric emptying. One approach uses electrogastrography before and after a provocative water load test. Patients ingest water until they feel 'full' within a 5-minute period. Gastric myoelectrical activity is recorded and analyzed before and after the water load. EGGs and the amount of water ingested are reproducible and objective measures. Other test meals or drugs may be given during EGG recordings. Gastric dysrhythmias are found in 30–58% of patients with functional dysmotility-like dyspepsia.

After mucosal and structural disorders are excluded (Figure 6.4, Step 1), gastric neuromuscular disorders should be considered as diagnostic possibilities (Figure 6.4, Step 2). As shown in Figure 6.4, if a gastric dysrhythmia is diagnosed with the EGG test, then the patient has a gastric neuromuscular disorder. Some of these patients (approximately 20%) will also have gastroparesis. Prokinetic therapy with metoclopramide, bethanechol or domperidone (or cisapride if available) is appropriate for patients with gastric dysrhythmias. If further characterization of the gastric neuromuscular disorder is desirable, then a solid-phase gastric emptying test may be performed to document the presence or absence of gastroparesis. In some centers, an antroduodenal manometry test is performed to further diagnose the neuromuscular abnormalities.

On the other hand, if the patient with unexplained dyspepsia symptoms has a normal EGG, then visceral hypersensitivity or non-gastric causes of the symptoms should be considered (Figure 6.4). Most patients with functional dyspepsia ingest lower than normal volumes of water as part of the water load test (approximately 300 mL versus 600 mL in control subjects). Thus, one approach is to treat these patients with drugs such as amitriptyline (although controlled trials are not available), fedotozine or sumatriptan. A gastric emptying study can also be considered in these patients. Gastroparesis with normal EGG test suggests either electromechanical dissociation or gastric outlet obstruction. Gastric outlet obstruction is a possibility if uniformly high-amplitude 3 cpm waves are present. The barostat test is used in some motility centers to quantify fundic tone and visceral sensitivity.

Finally, patients with persistent dyspepsia symptoms and normal EGG with normal water load may have non-gastric causes for their symptoms. In these patients, the diagnoses of atypical GERD, gallbladder disease and irritable bowel syndrome (IBS) should be considered or reconsidered. CNS disorders should be excluded in the patient with persistent nausea or intermittent vomiting, but usually other neurological findings are present. Thus, further testing in these patients with normal endoscopy and EGG tests should be considered. A 24-hour pH study, gallbladder-emptying study, computerized axiotomography of the brain, or an electroencephalogram may be proposed, depending on clinical circumstances.

To recap, in order to place diagnosis and treatment on a pathophysiological basis, this approach to the patient with persistent dyspepsia symptoms encompasses Step 1 testing to diagnose mucosal or structural diseases, and Step 2 testing to diagnose gastric neuromuscular disorders. According to the results of the EGG and gastric emptying tests carried out in Step 2, four pathophysiological categories are defined as shown in Figure 6.6. As described below, treatment can be designed or further diagnostic tests can be considered for the patients in these categories.

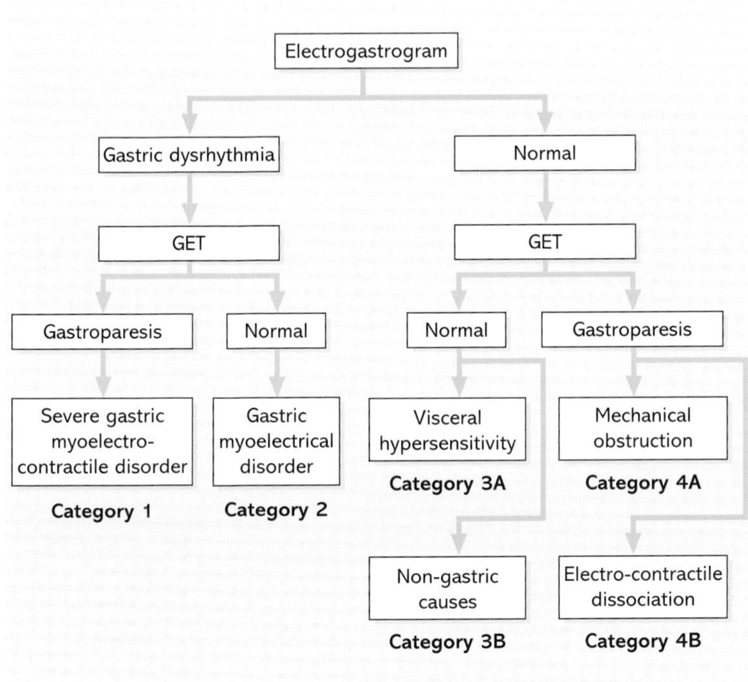

Figure 6.6 Categories of gastric neuromuscular dysfunction can be defined by electrogastrogram with water-load test and gastric emptying test (GET) results in patients with unexplained dyspepsia symptoms.

Category 1: gastric dysrhythmia and gastroparesis. The presence of gastric dysrhythmia and gastroparesis provides evidence of a diffuse and severe electrocontractile disorder of the stomach. The causes of the gastroparesis must be reviewed (see Table 6.1). Common diagnoses in this category are diabetes mellitus, post-surgical gastroparesis and idiopathic gastroparesis.

Category 2: gastric dysrhythmias and normal gastric emptying. The presence of a gastric dysrhythmia indicates abnormal myoelectrical activity of the stomach, but the myoelectrical abnormality is not severe enough to affect overall gastric emptying rate. The gastric dysrhythmia is believed to have a role in the generation of the dysmotility-like symptoms, particularly nausea. The mechanisms that generate gastric dysrhythmias range from decreased vagal activity to increased sympathetic neural activity. Injury to the enteric neurons or gastric smooth muscle cells may be present. Loss of or damage to interstitial cells of Cajal are also possible pathophysiological mechanisms for gastric dysrhythmias. Correction of gastric dysrhythmias with prokinetic agents such as metoclopramide or domperidone is associated with improvement in symptoms.

Category 3: normal gastric electrical activity and normal gastric emptying. These patients have no evidence of contractile or electrical abnormalities of the stomach. Visceral hypersensitivity of the stomach should be considered (Category 3A). These patients frequently ingest lower than normal volumes of water, indicating a hypersensitivity to stretch of the gastric wall even if gastric dysrhythmias are not present. The other possibility is that the symptoms reflect non-gastric diseases and disorders (Category 3B). Patients in Category 3B also have normal electrical rhythm and emptying, but symptoms are due to non-gastric disorders such as atypical GERD, delayed gallbladder emptying, irritable bowel syndrome, or CNS disorders.

Category 4: normal gastric electrical activity and gastroparesis. When the EGG signal is an unvarying and high-amplitude 3 cpm pattern, then mechanical obstruction should be considered (Category 4A). On the other hand, if there is normal-amplitude 3 cpm EGG activity, then there is a possibility of electrocontractile dissociation (Category 4B).

Treatment

With a specific diagnosis, more directed or aggressive therapy can be provided. For example, if the 24-hour esophageal pH study shows that frequent acid-reflux episodes are associated with symptoms, either a more aggressive approach to acid suppression can be initiated or prokinetic therapy started. If the major pathological finding is delayed gallbladder emptying and if other possibilities have been excluded, cholecystectomy may relieve symptoms. Similarly, once a diagnosis is made on the basis of gastric emptying and dysrhythmia, several different therapeutic options are available.

Drug therapy. Patients with gastroparesis and gastric dysrhythmia have severe gastric neuromuscular dysfunction and may require aggressive treatment with gastric prokinetic or combination therapy. Sufferers should be given a realistic expectation of the benefits that they are likely to experience with this kind of treatment.

Very few drugs are available currently to treat functional dyspepsia (Table 6.4). If the symptoms are ulcer-like, more aggressive acid-suppressant therapy may be tried. For dysmotility-like dyspepsia symptoms the following may be given: metoclopramide, 10–20 mg four times a day; cisapride, 10–20 mg four times a day; or domperidone, 10–20 mg four times a day. Prokinetic drugs generally reduce functional dyspepsia symptoms more effectively than H_2-receptor antagonists or placebo. The macrolide antibiotic erythromycin stimulates antral contractility and improves the gastric emptying rate.

Combination prokinetic therapy has not been well studied; it should probably be given in consultation with a gastroenterologist because of the risk of potentially adverse interactions. Drug studies that focus on one or two predominant dyspepsia symptoms, such as bloating or nausea, have not been performed, thus drugs must be tried empirically.

Metoclopramide is a D_2-receptor antagonist in the brain and stomach. It also stimulates acetylcholine release from the myenteric neurons and has some 5-HT_3 receptor antagonist activity. Metoclopramide is an anti-emetic and gastric prokinetic drug.

Side-effects. Metoclopramide is associated with central nervous system side-effects. These include:

TABLE 6.4

Treatment of functional dyspepsia

Agent	Rationale
Ulcer-like dyspepsia	
H_2-receptor antagonist	• Acid sensitivity
Proton-pump inhibitor	• Acid sensitivity
Dysmotility-like dyspepsia	
Cisapride*	• Acetylcholine deficit
Metoclopramide	• ?Dopamine excess • ?Acetylcholine deficit
Erythromycin	• Motilin receptor not stimulated
Domperidone**	• ?Dopamine excess
Fedotozine (not available in the UK/USA)	• ?Opiate pathway dysfunction

*Available only via compassionate clearance protocols (USA).
**Not approved for use in USA

- depression
- confusion
- mental-status changes
- tardive dyskinesia.

Overall, 20–30% of patients taking metoclopramide will experience one or more side-effects that increase with higher doses.

Cisapride releases acetylcholine from the myenteric plexus, stimulating contractions in the small bowel and colon as well as the stomach. This can result in abdominal cramps and diarrhea. Cisapride also competes with other prescription drugs for the liver enzyme cytochrome P450 3A4. As a result, increased blood levels of cisapride may occur. High blood levels of cisapride may result in prolonged QT and ventricular dysrhythmia. Cisapride has been withdrawn in the USA and is available only via compassionate

Effect	Mechanism
• Acid suppression	• H_2-receptor blockade
• Acid suppression	• H^+/K^+ ATPase inhibitor
• Increased gastric contractions • Decreased gastric dysrhythmia	• Increased acetylcholine release by 5-HT_4 agonist
• Increased gastric contractions	• Dopamine antagonist (central and peripheral) • Increased acetylcholine release
• Increased gastric contractions	• Motilin receptor agonist
• Increased gastric contractions • Decreased gastric dysrhythmia	• Dopamine antagonist (peripheral)
• ?Decreased visceral sensitivity	• Kappa agonist

clearance protocols.

Domperidone is associated with increases in prolactin levels and a 5–10% incidence of prolactin-related side-effects, such as breast tenderness.

Erythromycin is a motilin agonist. Stimulation of motilin receptors on the antrum results in strong antral contractions. Erythromycin is associated with abdominal cramps, nausea and vomiting, and is not tolerated by many patients with functional dyspepsia.

Dietary therapy. Patients may find considerable benefit in modifying their diet. In the presence of gastric electrical and contractile abnormalities, the volume of food ingested should be reduced so that six smaller meals are consumed during the day, rather than three main meals. The patient should be encouraged to snack frequently, so that larger volumes of liquid or solid foods do not stimulate dyspeptic symptoms by overly stretching fundus, corpus or antrum. A three-step diet for patients with nausea and vomiting has been suggested (Table 6.5).

Patients who cannot tolerate oral intake, are losing weight and are undernourished may need a gastrostomy tube for venting to prevent vomiting episodes and a jejunostomy for enteral feeding to maintain nutritional intake and weight stability.

Non-drug therapies. Several non-drug therapies are in development. They include acustimulation or acupuncture to relieve chronic nausea. For severe, drug-refractory nausea and vomiting due to gastroparesis, gastric pacemaking and gastric electrical stimulation devices have reduced symptoms and improved gastric dysrhythmia and gastric-

TABLE 6.5

A three-step diet for patients with nausea and vomiting*

Symptoms	Recommended foods
Severe	• Liquids such as: – commercial sports drinks with glucose, salt and potassium bouillon • Daily vitamin supplement
Less severe	• Foods such as: – soups with noodles or rice, crackers – some candies/confectionery • Daily vitamin supplement
Relatively mild	• Solid foods such as: – noodles – rice – potatoes – white meat • Daily vitamin supplement

*Modified from Koch 2000

emptying rates in small numbers of selected patients. These exciting non-drug therapies appear promising, and clinical research will indicate the settings in which these therapeutic modalities are appropriate.

Functional dyspepsia – Key points

- Pathophysiological mechanisms underlying dysmotility-like dyspepsia symptoms range from gastric dysrhythmias to gastroparesis.
- Electrogastrography and gastric emptying tests are non-invasive tests to diagnose gastric neuromuscular disorders.
- Dietary counseling and drug and non-drug therapies are used to improve gastric neuromuscular function and meal-related dyspepsia symptoms.

Key references

Brzana RJ, Bingaman S, Koch KL. Gastric myoelectrical activity in patients with gastric outlet obstruction and idiopathic gastroparesis. *Am J Gastroenterol* 1998;93:1083–9.

Cucchiara S, Minella R, Riezzo G et al. Reversal of gastric electrical dysrhythmias by cisapride in children with functional dyspepsia: report of three cases. *Dig Dis Sci* 1992;37:1136–40.

Gilja OH, Hausken T, Wilhelmsen I, Berstad A. Impaired accommodation of proximal stomach to a meal in functional dyspepsia. *Dig Dis Sci* 1996;41:689–96.

Koch KL. Dyspepsia of unknown origin. Pathophysiology, diagnosis and treatment. *Dig Dis* 1997;15:316–29.

Koch KL. Therapy of nausea and vomiting. In: Wolfe MM, ed. *Therapy of Digestive Disorders*. Philadelphia:WB Saunders, 2000:731–46.

Koch KL, Hong S-P, Xu L. Reproducibility of gastric myoelectrical activity and the water load test in patients with dysmotility-like dyspepsia symptoms and in control subjects. *J Clin Gastroenterol* 2000;31:125–9.

Koch KL, Stern RM, Stewart WR et al. Gastric emptying and gastric myoelectrical activity in patients with symptomatic diabetic gastroparesis: effects of long-term domperidone treatment. *Am J Gastroenterol* 1988;84:1069–75.

Laine L, Schoenfeld P, Fennerty MB. Therapy for *Helicobacter pylori* in patients with non-ulcer dyspepsia. A meta-analysis of randomized, controlled trials. *Ann Intern Med* 2001;134:361–9.

Parkman HP, Miller MA, Trate D et al. Electrogastrography and gastric emptying scintigraphy are complementary for assessment of dyspepsia. *J Clin Gastroenterol* 1997;24:214–19.

Stanghellini V, Tosetti C, Paternico A et al. Risk indicators of delayed gastric emptying of solids in patients with functional dyspepsia. *Gastroenterology* 1996;110:1036–42.

Stanghellini V, Tosetti C, Paternico A et al. Predominant symptoms identify different subgroups in functional dyspepsia. *Am J Gastroenterol* 1999;94:2080–5.

Tack J, Caenepeel P, Fischler B et al. Symptoms associated with hypersensitivity to gastric distention in functional dyspepsia. *Gastroenterology* 2001;121:526–35.

Talley NJ, Stanghellini V, Heading RC et al. Functional gastroduodenal disorders: *Gut* 1999;45(suppl. 2):II37–42.

7 Future trends

Towards safer NSAID therapy

Traditional NSAIDs are associated with a substantial incidence of serious gastrointestinal adverse events. If Cox-2 specific agents are adopted as a first-line therapy it is reasonable to predict that there will be a decline in the incidence of drug-induced ulcer disease (see Chapter 4).

An alternative approach to safer NSAID therapy is to link the anti-inflammatory drug to a nitric oxide-donating agent. Local nitric oxide production appears to protect the gastroduodenal mucosa, but results of human studies are not yet available.

Towards more cost-effective control of *H. pylori*

The incidence of *H. pylori* infection and associated diseases has declined in industrialized countries during the past 30 years, largely due to improved hygiene and living standards. We can predict that, as similar changes take place in the developing world, the same trend will also be seen in these countries. Nevertheless, a more effective means of controlling and eradicating the infection than is currently available would be a major contribution to world health.

Future antibiotics. The genomic sequence of *H. pylori* is now known, and this has provided the means of identifying which of its genes are essential for viability. The products of such genes include those necessary for the synthesis of nucleic acids and proteins, particularly those involved in maintaining the integrity of cell membranes. Recombinant gene technology will facilitate the production of these proteins for use in studies that will, in turn, enable highly specific 'antibiotic' drugs to be developed.

Vaccination. Although it may prove possible to eradicate *H. pylori* in the future with target-specific drugs, worldwide control of the infection is likely to depend on the development of a vaccine. In most circumstances, a vaccine is given prophylactically to uninfected people to produce antibodies that prevent clinical infection on subsequent contact with the organism. This may well prove possible in respect of *H. pylori*. However, universal preventive vaccination may not be cost-effective, even in the developed world.

An alternative is 'therapeutic immunization', which involves vaccinating those already infected to boost the host response to a level that leads to eradication. Experiments in mice and ferrets have been successful, but it will be several years before a product is available commercially. Nevertheless, immunization of serologically screened subjects with this type of vaccine might be more feasible and cost-effective than universal prophylactic vaccination or antibiotic therapy.

Towards more effective control of ulcer bleeding

There will be an increasing usage of endoscopic therapeutic techniques for the management of acute peptic ulcer bleeding. The efficacy of adrenaline or sclerosant injection and thermal modalities has now been established and promises to reduce the need for surgery, especially in high-risk elderly and frail patients.

Towards improved diagnosis and treatment of GERD

Increasingly, proton-pump inhibitors will become the basic treatment for typical heartburn due to GERD. Patients with GERD and symptoms of gastric dysmotility (GERD plus) will be recognized as a distinct patient subgroup and given combination therapy with proton-pump inhibitors and prokinetic agents. Also, atypical symptoms of GERD will be better understood, properly diagnosed and effectively treated. These developments will have a significant impact on the diagnosis and treatment of disorders such as asthma, aspiration pneumonia, chronic cough and hoarseness.

As the cost of endoscopy decreases in the USA, a greater number of patients with chronic heartburn symptoms will undergo this procedure to establish the presence or absence of Barrett's epithelium. However, tests to identify at-risk patients are needed to ensure endoscopies are only performed on appropriate patient populations. This may lead to a decreasing incidence of esophageal cancer.

Continually improving laparoscopic surgical techniques will make surgery an option for more patients with drug-refractory heartburn or atypical symptoms of GERD. Appropriate pre-operative evaluation of esophageal and gastric motility will be an increasingly important consideration for these patients to ensure optimal surgical outcome. Endoscopic procedures for GERD have been approved in the USA and appear to be efficacious. Open or laparascopic operations can be avoided, but long-term studies are ongoing for radiofrequency ablation therapy and endoscopic plication procedures for patients with GERD.

Future investigations into the pathophysiology of GERD may reveal new mechanisms that will lead to the development of new treatments. Improved therapy based on the known mechanisms of GERD, such as transient lower esophageal sphincter relaxations, will also become a reality. The relevance of other agents injurious to the esophageal mucosa, such as bile acids, pancreatic juices and *H. pylori*, will be clarified further.

Towards improved diagnosis and treatment of functional dyspepsia

At present, functional dyspepsia is a rather ill-defined clinical area. Our understanding of the pathophysiology and treatment of dyspepsia is improving, thus clarifying the meaning of the term. 'Functional dyspepsia' has little meaning for patients and is poorly defined in the minds of most physicians. Indeed, it will probably be abandoned altogether with time. In the future, it is possible that the pathophysiological mechanisms involved in the condition will be shown not to be functional, but in fact neuromuscular and/or hormonal.

The pathophysiological mechanisms of nausea and bloating will be clearly defined in coming years, allowing the development of new and more specific medical and non-medical treatments. Specific drugs for abnormal fundic, antral or pyloric tone will be available. Specific anti-arrhythmic drugs for tachygastrias or bradygastrias will be developed. Gastric pacemaker therapy is already a research reality for severe gastroparesis, nausea and vomiting. Acustimulation, acupuncture and herbal medicines may also be used more often to treat these symptoms in mild to moderately severe gastric neuromuscular disorders.

Controlled trials will allow for rational choice of these non-traditional treatments.

Understanding of the parasympathetic and sympathetic afferent nervous system pathways that carry information from peripheral organs in the gastrointestinal system to the central nervous system, where inflammation or neuromuscular/hormonal dysfunction is perceived as noxious sensations, such as nausea, fullness and bloating, will be important. New classes of treatment will be developed to modulate such vagal and sympathetic nervous system afferent neural traffic.

Useful addresses

American Gastroenterological Association
7910 Woodmont Avenue, 7th floor
Bethesda, MD 20814, USA
phone: 301 654 2055
fax: 301 652 3890
www.gastro.org

British Society of Gastroenterology
3 St Andrew's Place, Regent's Park
London NW1 4LB, UK
phone: 020 7387 3534
fax: 020 7487 3734
www.bsg.org.uk
bsg@mailbox.ulcc.ac.uk

Digestive Disorders Foundation
3 St Andrew's Place
London NW1 4LB, UK
www.digestivediseases.org.uk
[information on GI disease for the public]

Cancer BACUP
3 Bath Place, Rivington Street
London EC2A 3JR, UK
Counselling 0141 553 1553
Information 0808 800 1234
[information on cancer for the public]

The Helicobacter Foundation
www.helico.com

The Coeliac Society UK
PO Box 220, High Wycombe
Bucks HP11 2HY, UK
phone: 01494 437238
fax: 01494 474349
www.coeliac.co.uk

National Electronic Library for Health (UK)
www.nelh.nhs.uk

Cochrane Library
www.nelh.nhs.uk/cochrane.asp

Medline
www.ncbi.alm.nih.gov/entrez/query.fcgi

Medical Matrix
www.medicalmatrix.org/reg/login.asp
[database for health-care professionals]

Doctor online
www.doctoronline.nhs.uk
[general search engine]

Medicdirect
www.medicdirect.co.uk
[for patients and support groups]

Mirago Health UK
www.medisearch.co.uk
[search engine for patients]

Index